TESTIMONI/

M000250037

TO WHOM IT MAY CONCERN

RE: Dr. Rao Konduru's Publications:
    Reversing Obesity
    Reversing Sleep Apnea
    Reversing Insomnia

    Dr. Rao Konduru, PhD is a patient of mine who has suffered from chronic diabetes for most of his life; He also suffered from uncontrollable obesity, sleep apnea and chronic insomnia for the past 3 to 4 years. He has managed to reverse all of these conditions by taking non-pharmacological and science-based natural measures with great success. He has created 3 how-to user guides/books with regard to how he achieved this, and I recommend these books for anyone suffering from these conditions.

Sincerely,

Dr. Ali Ghahary, MD
Brentwood Medical Clinic
Burnaby, British Columbia, Canada

This book "Reversing Obesity" will make you THIN in a matter of days by simply following the easy-to-understand rapid weight-loss instructions and the do-it-yourself recipes illustrated by Dr. RK. When the stubborn fat around his belly refused to melt away, Dr. RK took a wise decision. He very carefully jotted down all kinds of junk foods he had been eating here and there, every now and then. By exercising self-discipline and high willpower, he completely eliminated all those junk foods from his whole foods diet. Voila, the results were astounding! He started losing weight quickly as the stubborn fat melted away day-by-day right in front of his eyes. He explains how healthy whole foods are, and at the same time how harmful processed foods and refined foods are, and how to avoid them in order to achieve successful weight-loss results.

If you are obese or overweight, this book is a must-read to achieve rapid weight-loss results and to reverse many health disorders and diseases, including type 2 diabetes, sleep apnea and chronic insomnia.

 - Prime Publishing Co.
New Westminster, British Columbia, Canada

This book "Reversing Obesity" isn't just any guide to miraculous weight loss. It is a compilation of hard-hitting facts, meticulous details and extraordinary results. It is the true and inspiring story of Dr. RK who succeeded in reversing his obesity permanently.

Healthy eating habits are necessary if one wants to lose weight and live well. In his book, Dr. RK teaches us simple, healthy and easy-to-make recipes using whole foods only. In addition, his weight-loss tips are extremely useful to implement the plan.

Dr. RK is a living example of a successful weight loss plan; a plan that helped him accomplish an absolute reversal of obstructive sleep apnea and chronic insomnia. After losing over 40 pounds of excess body weight more than a year back, he has maintained normal body weight until today, which is yet another achievement. This book has all the clues to not just rapid weight loss, but also on how to maintain normal weight after shedding off those extra pounds.

In my opinion, this book is the best thing that could ever happen to obese and overweight people. Only reading it could tell you why.

- Ms. Muriel D'Souza, Advertising Copywriter, Vancouver, British Columbia, Canada

----

Reversing Obesity

Self-Discovered Weight-Loss Method Illustrated

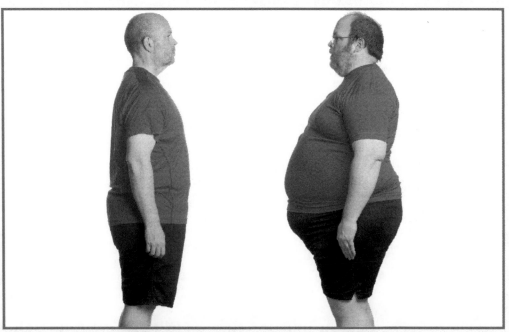

**After Losing 40 Pounds and 12 Inches Around the Waist,
Dr. RK Reversed His Obstructive Sleep Apnea!
Dr. RK Carefully Explained His Weight-Loss Method In This Book!**

LEARN HOW TO

- Recognize Whole Foods, Processed Foods & Refined Foods!
- Prepare Pre-Workout & Post-Workout Meals With Whole Foods!
- Eliminate Processed Foods & Refined Foods from Your Meals!
- Count Calories Using the Measuring Cups or by Weighing!
- Find Out the Amount of Fat, Protein & Carbs in Any Meal!
- Exercise (Walking/Gym Workout) Daily to Promote Weight Loss!
- Monitor the Body Mass Index (BMI) Every Week!
- Consume Apple Cider Vinegar: Appetite Suppressant, Digestion Promoter!
- Drink Purified Water, 8 to 16 Cups Per day!
- Very Important, Yet Powerful Weight-Loss Tips Included!

This Guide Will Make You A Self-Taught Weight-Loss Expert!

Rao Konduru, PhD

FOREWORD

Losing weight is an art. But if you are not artistic about it, you may end up regaining all the weight you've lost, even if you are workout savvy or a fitness guru. Many people lose weight working hard in the gym, but regain all the pounds they've burned within a few months just because of the lack of self-discipline.

If you are accustomed to eating out in restaurants, no matter how hard you workout in the gym, the fat in your belly increases unstoppably. Many of the restaurant foods are made from processed foods and refined foods. Processed foods are manufactured by adding preservatives, artificial colors and flavors including salt (sodium), monosodium glutamate (MSG), hydrogenated oils, fillers, sugars and sweeteners for a longer shelf life in the supermarkets. Refined foods, mostly carbohydrates could trigger your food cravings, similar to the urge drug addicts experience. Carbohydrates spike blood sugar levels demanding increased insulin production from pancreas, which could in turn result in type 2 diabetes. A typical example is the white flour or all purpose white flour made from grains (mostly wheat, rice or both). The altered texture and flavor make the body crave more of it. That is why your body wants more and more processed foods and refined foods and manufactures fat in the belly.

JUNK FOODS are strategically manufactured using processed foods and refined foods, adding large quantities of sugar, salt, oil, fat and several other chemicals including artificial colors and flavors to boost our cravings, so we buy more and eat more. Junk foods sabotage our weight-loss efforts.

By consuming whole foods and at the same time eliminating processed foods and refined foods from your diet, you can very easily transform your body's functionality within a few days, and even feel good about your health in general. You can see results within days, and feel a lot better. The cravings for processed foods and refined foods can be abolished by tasting whole foods in every meal you consume throughout the day. Consuming whole foods is an easy task, but avoiding processed foods and refined foods is the most difficult task for many people. If you are wise enough, you could develop a meal plan by restricting your diet to whole foods only, and you could be a winner in the weight loss plan.

After losing 40 pounds of body weight and 12 inches around the waist, Dr. RK reversed his obstructive sleep apnea successfully. It is almost a year after he did so, and until now he hasn't regained a pound back. As a matter of fact, he has even lost another 5 pounds during the past year. His strategy is: "Just consume the whole foods only and strictly avoid the processed foods and refined foods by exercising high self-discipline." He has carefully explained his method in this book "Reversing Obesity."

Prime Publishing Co.

COPYRIGHT

Book Title: Reversing Obesity
Sub-Title: Self-Discovered Weight-Loss Diet Illustrated
Author: Rao Konduru, PhD (Also Called Dr. RK)
Address: 720 – Sixth Street, Unit: 171
    New Westminster, BC, Canada, V3L 3C5
Website: https://reversingobesity.ca/
ISBN #   ISBN 978-0-9731120-3-0

This book "Reversing Insomnia" has been registered under ISBN Number "ISBN 978-0-9731120-3-0" with the National Library of Canada Cataloguing in Publication, Ottawa, Ontario, Canada. The original manuscript has been submitted to the Legal Deposits, Library and Archives Canada, Ottawa, Ontario, Canada.

DISCLAIMER: The author of this book titled "Reversing Obesity" assumes no liability or responsibility including, without limitation, incidental and consequential damages, personal injury or wrongful death resulting from the use of any treatment method presented in this book. Misusing the obesity treatment procedure could lead to serious side effects. More specifically, an extremely-low, daily calorie intake without appropriate caution and care could lead to nutritional deficiency or other health problems. All contents in this book are for educational purpose only, and do not in any way represent professional medical advice. A reader should seek appropriate medical advice when using the methods illustrated in this book.

TABLE OF CONTENTS

CHAPTER 1   MAIN ARTICLE
WEIGHT-LOSS DIET (LEVEL-I)
Daily Calorie Intake: 2000 Calories

INITIAL INSTRUCTIONS

1. This course is designed to teach you how to lose weight, and at the same time the author (Dr. RK) describes his own weight-loss experience so that you could learn from the techniques he has developed and the successful results he has achieved.

2. NOT TO WORRY if you are not food-label savvy or a calorie-counter. By following the simple instructions on cooking whole foods, by sticking to the measured amounts of foods and by using the easily-adaptable recipes presented in this course, you can lose weight and achieve the desired results. You should be faithful to your exercise and have the willpower and self-discipline to avoid processed and refined foods.

3. If you are curious about learning calorie-counting, then this course would teach you how to calculate calories of the meal on your dinner plate, and how find out the amount of fat, protein and carbohydrates in any meal. See Appendix-A for details.

4. You weigh the food items using an electronic balance and do the calorie-counting only on the first day when you prepare a meal, not every day.

5. After the first day, you stick to the same measuring cups to prepare a similar meal every day. You can add, remove or replace some food items in the meal using measuring cups. You can replace one vegetable with another, it won't change the calorie distribution of the total meal much. If you want to add or remove any meat, chicken, or fish to the meal of vegetables, then you need to do the calorie-counting again. It is better to stick to the same or similar kind of meals every day when you opt for a weight-loss program.

6. Approximate calorie-counting is necessary so that you can compare previously tried meal-plans with your current one, and make changes in order to increase or decrease the daily calorie consumption, fat content, protein content and carbohydrate content. By manipulating or by lowering the fat content, and by adjusting the daily protein consumption, you can make adequate changes to your diet, and lose weight.

7. When you buy a packaged food item, always check the label on that package or on the bottle for the nutritional information. If the label says, it has preservatives (high in sodium), artificial colors and flavors, do not buy and bring it home. Always try to buy and eat whole foods, and eliminate processed foods and refined foods from your meal. You should always keep in mind that you eat only complex carbohydrates, which are low in sugar with no refined flour, and avoid eating simple carbohydrates, which are high in sugar and contain a lot of refined flour.

8. Whenever you buy raw vegetables, fruits or other whole foods, find out their nutritional information from reliable sources like:
> a. The label of the package you've just purchased
> b. The FDA website (http://www.fda.gov/Food/)
> c. The USDA website (https://ndb.nal.usda.gov/ndb/search/list)
> d. Do a Google Search (for example type "calories broccoli")

9. Always remember (memorize and keep this info in mind): Fat has 9 calories/gm, Protein has 4 calories/gm and Carbohydrates have 4 calories/gm. Calories always imply Kcal (there is a misconception in the food industry).

8 am – 9 am   Breakfast (OPTION-1)

Do not consume heavy breakfast when resting at home.

Table 1.1 Recipe of breakfast (OPTION 1).

Food Item	Amount
Whole Wheat Pita Bread (1/2 Pita)	1/2 pita
Organic Coffee (10 g Brewed)	1 cup
2% Organic Milk (2 tbsp), No Sugar	2 tbsp

Table 1.2 Calories & nutritional information of the breakfast (OPTION 1).

Food Item	Weight (gm)	Calories	Protein (gm)	Fat (gm)	Carbo (gm)
Whole Wheat Pita Bread (1/2 Pita)	28.5	65	2.5	0.5	13.5
Organic Coffee (10 g Brewed)	10	4	0.28	0.05	0
2% Organic Milk (2 tbsp)	15	7	0.54	0.27	0.66
Total →	53.5	76	3.32	0.82	14.16
Calories calculated →		77.3	13.28	7.38	56.64
Percentage (%) →			17%	10%	73%

8 am – 9 am   Breakfast (OPTION-2)

Table 1.3 Recipe of the breakfast (OPTION 2).

Food Item	Amount
Organic Kamut Puffs	1 cup
Organic Almond Milk	1 cup
Organic Banana (Medium-size)	medium
Organic Coffee (10 g Brewed)	1 cup
2% Organic Milk (2 tbsp), No Sugar	2 tbsp

Table 1.4 Calories & nutritional information of the breakfast (OPTION 2).

Food Item	Weight (gm)	Calories	Protein (gm)	Fat (gm)	Carbo (gm)
Organic Kamut Puffs (1 Cup)	20	50	2	0	11
Organic Almond Milk (1 Cup)	250	60	1	2.5	8
Organic Banana (Medium-size)	130	110	1	0	30
Organic Coffee (10 g Brewed)	10	4	0.28	0.05	0
2% Organic Milk (2 tbsp)	15	7	0.54	0.27	0.66
Total →	425	231	4.82	2.82	49.66
Calories calculated →		243.3	19.28	25.38	198.64
Percentage (%) →			8%	10%	82%

11 am - 12 pm   Pre-Workout Meal: Egg-White Omelet with Veggies
It Could Be Your LUNCH / BRUNCH

Table 1.5   Recipe of the pre-workout meal (egg-white omelet with veggies).

Food Item/Ingredient	Amount
Egg White (extra large organic Eggs)	2
(98% of Egg Yolk is removed with a spoon)	
Broccoli (organic)	1 cup
Cauliflower (organic)	
(Replace this with Egg Plant/Other)	
Kale (organic)	1 cup
(Replace this with Spinach/Cilantro/Parsley/Other)	
Radishes (3 with stems)	3
(Replace this with your favorite vegetable)	
Bell Peppers (Red/Yellow/Green)	1/2 cup
Red Onion (organic)	1 cup
(Replace this with Yellow Onion)	
Ginger (fresh, peeled)	1/2 cup
Garlic (fresh, peeled, 4 cloves)	4 cloves
Sea Salt (a little bit)	A little
Curry Powder (organic)	1 tsp
Cayenne Pepper (organic)	1 tsp
Turmeric (organic root powder)	1/2 tbsp
Flaxseed (organic, ground)	1 spoon
Extra Virgin Olive Oil (a little)	A little
Purified Water (250 mL)	1 cup

Fresh vegetables (preferably organic) are washed thoroughly, without soaking, by submerging them in a basin filled with warm tap water and then dried using a salad dryer. The washed and dried vegetables are then cut into small pieces, and measured using the measuring cups before cooking.

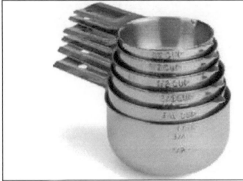

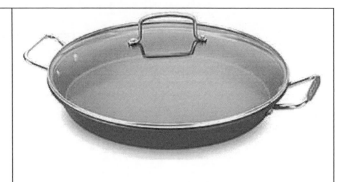

Figure 1.1 Measuring cups. (1 cup, 3/4 cup, 1/2 cup, 1/3 cup, 1/4 cup)	Figure 1.2 Non-stick fry pan/skillet with glass lid. (at least 10" in diameter)

Table 1.6 Calories & nutritional information of the pre-workout meal (egg-white omelet with veggies).

Food Item	Weight (gm)	Calories	Protein (gm)	Fat (gm)	Carbo (gm)
Egg White (2 Ex Large Organic Eggs)	94	50	10	0	0
(98% of Egg Yolk is removed with a spoon)					
Broccoli (Organic, 1 Cup)	80	26	2.5	0.30	4.7
Cauliflower (Organic, 1 Cup)	120	25	2.0	0	5.3
(Replace this with Egg Plant/Other)					
Kale (Organic, 1 Cup)	40	20	1.31	0.30	4
(Replace this with Spinach/Cilantro/Parsley/Other)					
Radishes (3 with stems)	60	10	0.42	0.06	2
(Replace this with your favorite vegetable)					
Bell Peppers (Red/Yellow/Green 1/2 Cup)	60	15	0.50	0	4
Red Onion (Organic, 1 Cup)	80	30	1	0.15	7
(Replace this with Yellow Onion)					
Ginger (Fresh, Peeled, 1/2 Cup)	60	30	0	0	6
Garlic (Fresh, Peeled, 4 cloves)	20	20	0	0	5.2
Sea Salt (a Little Bit)	2	0	0	0	0
Curry Powder (Organic, 1 tsp)	2	5	0	0	1
Cayenne Pepper (Organic, 1 tsp)	2	6	0	0	1
Turmeric (Organic Root Powder, 1/2 tbsp)	7	24	1	1	4
Flaxseed (Organic, Ground), 1 Spoon	15	70	3	5	0
Extra Virgin Olive Oil (A Little, 5 mL)	5	40	0	4.7	0
Purified Water (1 Cup=250 mL)	250	0	0	0	0
Total →	897	371	21.73	11.47	44.22
Calories calculated →		367.03	86.92	103.23	176.88
Percentage (%) →			23.68%	28.13%	48.19%

- All food items are weighed using an electronic balance on the first day only.
- All food items are prepared using the measuring cups from the second day onwards.
- Fat: 9 calories/gm; Protein: 4 calories/gm; Carbohydrates: 4 calories/gm.

PREPARATION: EGG-WHITE OMELET WITH VEGGIES

1. Wash all the organic vegetables by submerging them in a large basin filled with warm tap water (do not soak them). Then dry them using a salad dryer. Cut all the vegetables into small pieces, and place then in a large metal/glass bowl.

2. Crack two extra large organic eggs into another small metal/glass bowl. Try to scoop out at least 90% of the egg yolk. I was able to remove 98% of yolk without losing egg white.

3. Add the egg white to the vegetables with sea salt and all spices, and mix them thoroughly using a large spoon in the large bowl until all veggies are blended with egg white.

4. Place the non-stick pan or skillet of at least 10" diameter on the stove adjusted to medium heat. Drizzle only a little extra virgin olive oil so that the oil droplets cover most of the surface of the non-stick pan. There should be space between the droplets. The total amount of the extra virgin olive oil should not be more than a teaspoon. This is your total oil consumption per day. For the rest of the day, you don't consume more oil. If you experience any side effects such as itching, then you can consume a little more oil.

5. Pour the entire mixture of veggies and egg white onto the non-stick pan. When you do this, at first place the kale pieces all over the surface of the pan, and then place the remaining mixture on the top of the kale pieces so that it becomes easier to flip the omelet after it is cooked. Adjust the edges until you see the round shape of the omelet, then cover with a glass lid.

6. After 5 minutes of cooking, flip the omelet using a metal spatula and let it cook a few more minutes on the other side on low heat. Do not overcook the veggies (semi-cooked veggies are more nutritious). However you decide the right time of cooking depending on how you prefer the omelet.

7. When the omelet is cooked, place it on the dinner plate.

8. Once the omelet is cooked and ready, consume only the omelet without any side dish. Do not consume any side dishes such as bread, pan-fried potatoes, sausages or anything else. Drink at least a cup of purified water. You can also drink another cup of organic coffee if you like after you finish eating the omelet.

9. Then you exercise (either walk on the road or in the shopping mall or go to the gym and exercise). This omelet and the coffee are supposed to energize you and provide you with sufficient energy for an hour, and burn a lot more calories than you consumed. When you burn more calories than you consumed, you lose weight.

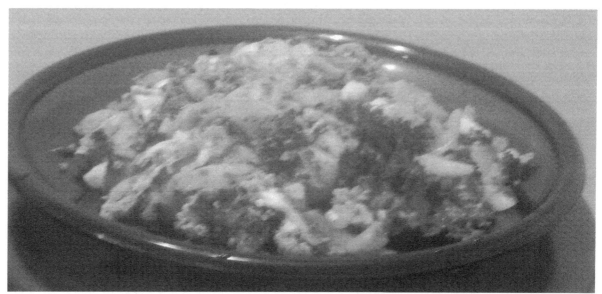

Figure 1.3 Egg-white omelet with 2 extra large organic eggs, veggies & spices.
It Contains 371 Calories, 22 g Protein, 11.5 g Fat and 44 g Carbs.

Egg-White Omelet is the most important meal of this weight-loss course. It does not look like a traditional omelet served in restaurants. It looks like a bunch of fried vegetables, but incorporated with egg white protein all over it. If you want to increase the amount of protein, add more egg white while cooking the omelet. This egg-white omelet contains very little salt and very little oil. By minimizing the salt consumption and oil consumption, you can lose weight fast. This omelet gives me energy to work out in the gym, and prevents me from hunger attacks throughout the day.

ADDITIONAL INSTRUCTIONS

10. IMPORTANT NOTE: Do not buy egg white being sold in packages in supermarkets. It is loaded with preservatives and it is high in sodium, which prevents weight loss.

11. Make your own egg white by cracking two or more extra large organic raw eggs. Discard the egg yolk or save it for other family members or for your pets. Do not lose egg white while removing the yolk. Try to keep 100% of egg white; it is a very important ingredient in this omelet. Wash your hands with soap after cracking the eggs and extracting the egg whites. Beware of Salmonella and take appropriate caution when you deal with eggs.

12. Egg yolk has high saturated fat & high cholesterol. You should not eat egg yolk every day. It is not good for weight loss. You can eat egg whites (which comprise 100% protein) every day. So try scooping out as much egg yolk as possible when you make the egg-white omelet.

13. Make your own egg-white omelet that suits your appetite. Choose your favorite vegetables and spices, and change the items every now and then. Eat a variety of vegetables every week so that your body gets all kinds of vitamins, minerals and fiber.

14. Don't be so precise about the amounts of the veggies when you use measuring cups. It is not a medicinal recipe, but it is an example of what I ate when I lost weight. If you don't feel full, feel free to add more veggies.

- Add a few more items you like such as mushrooms, basil, curry leaves, spinach, or other leafy vegetables not included here.
- Add more onions, bell peppers, fresh ginger, fresh garlic, etc.
- Add more spices such as mustard seeds, cumin seeds, sesame seeds, etc.

15. Find out the right quantities of veggies that suit your stomach and your appetite, and at the same time minimize the total quantity (total calories) of veggies, and be consistent while preparing the omelet every day. When you change the vegetables, add the same amounts by using the measuring cups.

16. Be consistent. Eat the same kind of egg-white omelet (pre-workout meal) every day. Maintain the same quantity (approximately the same calories). Have it at the same time of the day, just before exercising.

17. Continue with your weight-loss diet for at least 4 weeks to see if you have lost significant weight or inches on the waist. Monitor and record your weight and waist size every day. Maintain a weight-loss journal and make notes of everything you are doing. In 4 weeks, if you did not lose weight at all, then lower the daily calorie intake of the weight-loss diet by 500 calories, and proceed with your new diet for another 4 weeks, and so on.

18. The important thing that you should grasp is: You should not eat processed and refined foods while you are on the weight loss program. Instead, you should eat the same quantity of whole foods consistently every day by cooking them at home. Enforce a law on yourself so that you don't go out and eat processed foods or any kind of junk foods or sugary drinks at restaurants. By eating whole foods cooked at home and by drinking purified water, you can lose weight. So follow all the weight-loss tips (described at the end of this course) carefully.

19. **How To Minimize Salt Consumption & Oil Consumption**

Too much salt consumption and too much oil consumption prevent weight loss.

I minimized my salt consumption and oil consumption by using the following spice bottles for sea salt and oil.

SALT BOTTLE (on the left): Choose a spice bottle with small holes that would sprinkle only a tiny bit of salt onto the vegetables.

OIL BOTTLE (on the right): Choose a spice bottle with a few holes in the cap. If it has too many holes, close the holes in the cap by drilling the sandwich bag tags that are cut in short into the unwanted holes, leaving only 3 holes. This kind of bottle dispenses very little extra virgin olive oil onto the non-stick pan, when you make your egg-white omelet every day as the pre-workout meal. This is how you minimize your oil consumption.

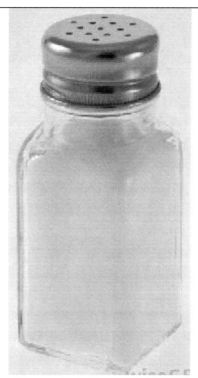

Figure 1.4 Sea salt bottle.
It has very tiny holes in the cap.

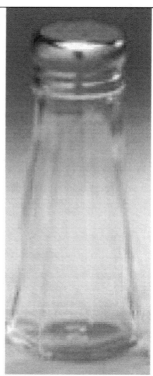

Figure 1.5 Extra virgin olive oil bottle.
It has only 3 tiny holes in the cap.

20. **EXERCISE EVERY DAY (If You Want to Lose Weight Fast)**

Make your own schedule for exercise, depending on your free time. Maintain the same schedule every day for eating meals and for exercise so that your body can easily adapt to your activities.

a. You can go out and walk on the road for an hour (if you don't have lower-leg pain or plantar fasciitis).
b. You can go to a large shopping mall and walk for an hour if the mall allows.
c. You can go to a local gym every day and exercise for 1 hour or more.

21. **HIGH-INTENSITY EXERCISE:** If you are capable, then go ahead and do a high-intensity exercise such as running on a treadmill at high speeds and with a high incline, elliptical, recumbent bike, upright bike, strength training, weight lifting, dumbbells, chest press, leg press, leg curl, upper-body pulldown and others. Monitor and record how many calories you burn every day. Record-keeping would help you compare and improve your workout performance, and thus you can maximize your ability to burn calories. Don't listen to people in the gym who say, "Don't record calories; they are not accurate."

22. **CONSUME MORE FOOD, BY ADDING OVEN-BAKED CHICKEN, FISH OR MEAT, WHEN YOU DO HIGH-INTENSITY EXERCISE EVERY DAY:** If you can do high intensity exercises, you can burn a lot more fat calories, and so you will need to eat more food or you could face hunger attacks. You can add organic chicken or meat to the egg white omelet (pre-workout meal) and increase the total daily calorie consumption in that case.

23. When I was much younger 5 years ago, 7 years ago and 10 years ago, I used to lose all the excess weight (35 pounds) simply through a high-intensity treadmill workout of 4 to 6 weeks, without having to watch my diet. But during the last 5 years, I have developed plantar fasciitis and lower-leg pain because of which I am unable to do high intensity exercise. So, I developed a low-calorie and low-fat whole food diet. I still use the treadmill at low speeds and the bike at a low level. But since I cannot do high intensity exercises, I decided to cut down on my diet. Now my experience tells me that the diet is more responsible for my weight loss than exercise.

+++
12:30 pm – 2 pm   **Exercise in the Gym**
                  After Eating the Pre-Workout Meal (Egg-White Omelet)

I go to gym every day (7 days a week), and exercise 60 to 90 minutes.
a. I do stretching, foam roller, sit ups on the inclined ab bench, upper-body pulldown, chest press, leg press, etc. for 20 to 30 min.

b. I then walk on the treadmill at a low speed and high incline for 30 minutes, Treadmill with Hill Program: Inclination varies between 5.5 and 11.3; Speed stays at 3 mph. Calories burned in a typical day with treadmill = 540 Kcal/hour.

c. After that I do recumbent bike for another 30 minutes (at Level 3).

d. During the exercise I drink 2 cups of purified water, which I carry with me.

I then go home and eat my post-workout meal, which I prepare before I go to the gym. See below in the next page for the post-workout meal.

++

2 pm – 3 pm   Post-Workout Meal (OPTION-1)
Rotisserie Chicken, Brown Rice & Vegetables

Table 1.7 Recipe of the post-workout meal (OPTION-1).

Food Item/Ingredient	Amount
Rotisserie Chicken Breast	1 Cup
Brown Rice (1/4 Cup Dry, 1 Cup Cooked)	1 Cup
Boiled Kidney Beans/Chickpeas	1/2 Cup
Cucumbers (Organic, Fresh)	1/2 Cup
Tomato (Organic, Fresh)	3/4 Cup
Sea Salt (Very Little)	Little
Cayenne Pepper (Organic, 1 tsp)	1 tsp
Extra Virgin Olive Oil (Petrelli) 5 mL	Little
Lemon Juice (2 tsp) + Purified Water	1 Cup

• Fresh cucumbers and fresh tomatoes are added to the meal using the measuring cups.

Table 1.8 Calories & nutritional information of the post-workout meal (OPTION-1).

Food Item	Weight (gm)	Calories	Protein (gm)	Fat (gm)	Carbo (gm)
Rotisserie Chicken Breast(1 Cup)	100	148	29	4	0
Brown Rice (1/4 Cup Dry, 1 Cup Cooked)	45	150	3	1.5	35
Boiled Kidney Beans.Chickpeas (1/2 Cup)	90	114	7.8	0.45	20.5
Cucumbers (Organic, Fresh, 1/2 Cup)	100	16	0.6	0.1	3.6
Tomato (Organic, Fresh, 3/4 Cup)	100	20	1	0.2	4.25
Sea Salt (Very Little)	2	0	0	0	0
Cayenne Pepper (Organic, 1 tsp)	2	0	0	0	0
Extra Virgin Olive Oil (Petrelli) 5 mL	5	40	0	4.66	0
Lemon Juice (2 tsp) + Purified Water	30	8	0.2	0	2.8
Total →	474	496	41.6	10.91	66.15
Calories calculated →		529.19	166.4	98.19	264.6
Percentage (%) →			31.44%	18.55%	50.00%

• All food items are weighed using electronic balance on the first day only.
• All food items are prepared using the measuring cups from the second day onwards.
• Fat: 9 calories/gm; Protein: 4 calories/gm; Carbohydrate: 4 calories/gm.

PREPARATION: Make your own post-workout meal with whole foods (oven-baked chicken, fish or meat along with your favorite vegetables, beans and spices). Cook the items in advance, enough to last for a week. Store them in the fridge so that you can microwave them and eat the post-workout meal immediately after exercise. Be consistent and consume the same quantity of each item of the meal (approximately the same calories) every day with the help of the measuring cups. Change and eat a variety of vegetables & beans every day so that your body gets the required energy along with all kinds of vitamins, minerals and fiber from the food items being consumed.

2 pm – 3 pm   Post-Workout Meal (OPTION-2)
Cottage Cheese (High in Protein), Brown Rice, Vegetables & Beans

Table 1.9 Recipe of the post-workout meal (Option-2).

Food Item/Ingredient	Amount
Cottage Cheese Dry Curd (Dairyland)	1/2 Cup
Brown Rice (1/4 Cup Dry, 1 Cup Cooked)	1 Cup
Yams (Organic Boiled)	1/2 Cup
Butternut Squash (Organic, Boiled)	1/2 Cup
Green Peppers (Boiled)	1/2 Cup
Chicpeas/Garbanzo (Organic, Boiled)	1/2 Cup
Sea Salt (Very Little)	Little
Cayenne Pepper (Organic, 1 tsp)	1 tsp
Purified Water (1 Cup)	1 Cup

● All fresh vegetables are washed, dried and cut into small pieces, and then measured using the measuring cups before cooking.

Table 1.10 Calories & nutritional information of the post-workout meal (OPTION-2).

Food Item	Weight (gm)	Calories	Protein (gm)	Fat (gm)	Carbo (gm)
Cottage Cheese Dry Curd (Dairyland, 1/2 Cup)	125	110	22	0.5	2
Brown Rice (1/4 Cup Dry, 1 Cup Cooked)	45	150	3	1.5	35
Yams (Organic Boiled, 1/2 Cup)	50	58	0.74	0.07	13.84
Butternut Squash (Organic, Boiled 1/2 Cup)	50	14	0.95	0.2	2.8
Green Peppers (Boiled, 1/2 Cup)	50	10	0.42	0.08	2.3
Chicpeas/Garbanzo (Organic, Boiled, 1/2 Cup)	82	134	7.5	2	22.5
Sea Salt (Very Little)	2	0	0	0	0
Cayenne Pepper (Organic, 1 tsp)	2	0	0	0	0
Purified Water (1 Cup)	250	0	0	0	0
Total →	656	476	34.61	4.35	78.44
Calories calculated →		491.35	138.44	39.15	313.76
Percentage (%) →			28.18%	7.97%	63.86%

● All food items are weighed using an electronic balance on the first day only.
● All food items are prepared using the measuring cups from the second day onwards.
● Fat: 9 calories/gm; Protein: 4 calories/gm; Carbohydrates: 4 calories/gm.

PREPARATION: Make your own post-workout meal with whole foods (cottage cheese dry curd, brown rice along with your favorite vegetables, beans and spices). Cook the items in advance, enough to last for a week. Store them in the fridge so that you can microwave them and eat the post-workout meal immediately after exercise. Be consistent and consume the same quantity of each item of the meal (approximately the same calories) every day with the help of the measuring cups. Change and eat a variety of vegetables & beans every day so that your body gets the required energy along with all kinds of vitamins, minerals and fiber from the food items being consumed.

Cottage Cheese (Dry Curd) Is Good for Weight Loss

Cottage cheese (dry curd) is an excellent food item if you want to lose weight. Check the nutritional information of cottage cheese shown below. It has low calories, is very high in protein, low in fat (almost zero) and low in carbohydrates (zero carbohydrates) too. It is very similar to egg white, which is 100% protein. When you buy this item, make sure it is not the creamy cottage cheese, which is loaded with high sodium (too much salt prevents weight loss and could cause high blood pressure). Always look for "Cottage Cheese Dry Curd with Low Sodium" on the label before purchasing it. Although it comes under processed foods, it should be considered a whole food because of its nutritional protein-rich, low-fat, low-carb, low-sodium composition. Organic cottage cheese (low sodium) is not available in this area (Vancouver, BC, Canada) so make your own from organic 1% milk or 2% milk.

Cottage Cheese Dry Curd (Dairyland/Other)
A Very Important Food Item to Lose Weight.
An Excellent Source of Protein Without Fat (1/2 cup has 22 g of Protein)
High Protein, Little Fat (Zero), Little Carb (Zero), Low Sodium, Low Cholesterol

Nutrition Facts	
Serving Size: 1/2 cup (125 g)	
Amount Per Serving	
Calories from Fat 4.5 Calories 110	
% Daily Values*	
Total Fat 0.5g	1%
Saturated Fat 0.3g	2%
Cholesterol 10mg	3%
Sodium 15mg	1%
Total Carbohydrates 2g	1%
Dietary Fiber -	
Sugars 2g	
Protein 22g	
Contains Vitamins & Minerals	
Vitamin A 2% Vitamin C -	
Calcium 4% Iron 2%	

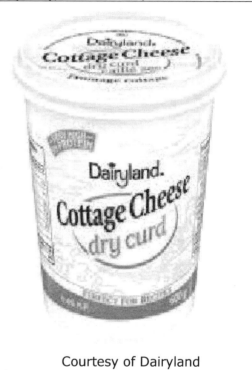

Courtesy of Dairyland
https://www.fatsecret.ca/calories-nutrition/dairyland/dry-curd-cottage-cheese/1-2-cup
Figure 1.6 Cottage cheese dry curd.

Make Your Own Cottage Cheese at Home from Organic 2% Milk:

Warm the 2% organic milk in a saucepan. Once it has reached lukewarm temperature, remove the saucepan from the heat. Add 1 to 2 tablespoons of organic apple cider vinegar and another tablespoon of lemon juice per a cup of warm 2% milk. Continue stirring until the warm 2% milk separates into a solid white mass and liquid whey. The solid white mass is the cottage cheese dry curd. Transfer the cottage cheese dry curd into a separate bowl. Do not discard the liquid whey as it has a lot of protein in it. Consume the cottage cheese dry curd (with the post-workout meal) as it is mostly protein. Use the liquid whey while cooking the vegetables or make a protein shake by blending it with organic fruits.

2 pm – 3 pm Post-Workout Meal (OPTION-3)
Cottage Cheese (high in protein), Boiled Vegetables & Beans

Table 1.11 Recipe of of the post-workout meal (OPTION-3).

Food Item/Ingredient	Amount
Cottage Cheese Dry Curd (Dairyland)	1/2 Cup
Egg White Ex Lg (Organic, Boiled, Without Yolk)	1 Egg
Carrots (Organic, Boiled)	1/2 Cup
Yams (Organic Boiled)	1/2 Cup
Butternut Squash (Organic, Boiled)	1/2 Cup
Green Peppers (Boiled)	1/2 Cup
Kidney Beans (Organic, Boiled)	1/2 Cup
Sea Salt (Very Little)	Little
Cayenne Pepper (Organic, 1 tsp)	1 tsp
Purified Water (1 Cup)	1 Cup

● All fresh vegetables are washed, dried and cut into small pieces, and then measured using the measuring cups before cooking.

Table 1.12 Calories & nutritional information of the post-workout meal (OPTION-3).

Food Item	Weight (gm)	Calories	Protein (gm)	Fat (gm)	Carbo (gm)
Cottage Cheese Dry Curd (Dairyland, 1/2 Cup)	125	110	22	0.5	2
Egg White Ex Lg (Organic, Boiled, Without Yolk)	47	25	5	0	0
Carrots (Organic, Boiled 1/2 Cup)	50	17	0.37	0.06	3.9
Yams (Organic Boiled, 1/2 Cup)	50	58	0.74	0.07	13.84
Butternut Squash (Organic, Boiled, 1/2 Cup)	50	14	0.95	0.2	2.8
Green Peppers (Boiled, 1/2 Cup)	50	10	0.42	0.08	2.3
Kidney Beans (Organic, Boiled 1/2 Cup)	90	114	7.8	0.45	20.5
Sea Salt (Very Little)	2	0	0	0	0
Cayenne Pepper (Organic, 1 tsp)	2	0	0	0	0
Purified Water (1 Cup)	250	0	0	0	0
Total →	716	348	37.28	1.36	45.34
Calories calculated →		342.72	149.12	12.24	181.36
Percentage (%) →			43.51%	3.57%	52.92%

PREPARATION: Make your own post-workout meal with whole foods (cottage cheese dry curd, brown rice along with your favorite vegetables, beans and spices). Cook the items in advance, enough to last for a week. Store them in the fridge so that you can microwave them and eat the post-workout meal immediately after exercise. Be consistent and consume the same quantity of each item of the meal (approximately the same calories) every day with the help of the measuring cups. Change and eat a variety of vegetables & beans every day so that your body gets the required energy along with all kinds of vitamins, minerals and fiber from the food items being consumed.

6 pm – 7 pm Evening Meal/Dinner (OPTION-1)
Baked Fish & Veggies

Table 1.13 Recipe of the evening meal/dinner (OPTION1).

Food Item	Amount
Salmon Fish (1 Fillet Baked, High Liner)	1 Fillet
Pre-Cooked Mixed Veggies (1/2 Cup) Great Value, Purchased at Walmart	1/2 Cup
Cucumbers (Organic, Fresh, 1/2 Cup)	1/2 Cup
Tomato (Organic, Fresh, 3/4 Cup)	3/4 Cup
Sea Salt (Very Little)	Little
Cayenne Pepper (Organic, 1 tsp)	1 tsp
Extra Virgin Olive Oil (Petrelli) 5 mL	Little
Lemon Juice (2 tsp) + Purified Water	1 Cup

● Fresh cucumbers and fresh tomatoes are added to the meal using the measuring cups.

Table 1.14 Calories & nutritional information of the evening meal/dinner (OPTION1).

Food Item	Weight (gm)	Calories	Protein (gm)	Fat (gm)	Carbo (gm)
Salmon Fish (1 Fillet Baked, High Liner)	110	130	21	1	0
Pre-Cooked Mixed Veggies (1/2 Cup) Great Value, Purchased at Walmart	50	50	2	1	11
Cucumbers (Organic, Fresh, 1/2 Cup)	100	16	0.6	0.1	3.6
Tomato (Organic, Fresh, 3/4 Cup)	100	20	1	0.2	4.25
Sea Salt (Very Little)	2	0	0	0	0
Cayenne Pepper (Organic, 1 tsp)	2	0	0	0	0
Extra Virgin Olive Oil (Petrelli) 5 mL	5	40	0	4.66	0
Lemon Juice (2 tsp) + Purified Water	30	8	0.2	0	2.8
Total →	399	264	24.8	6.96	21.65
Calories calculated →		248.44	99.2	62.64	86.6
Percentage (%) →			39.93%	25.21%	34.86%

● All food items are weighed using an electronic balance on the first day only.
● All food items are prepared using the measuring cups from the second day onwards.
● Fat: 9 calories/gm; Protein: 4 calories/gm; Carbohydrates: 4 calories/gm

PREPARATION: Make your own evening meal/dinner with whole foods (baked salmon fish, pre-cooked vegetables, fresh tomatoes, fresh cucumbers and spices). Be consistent and consume the same quantity of each item of the meal (approximately the same calories) every day with the help of the measuring cups. Change and eat a variety of vegetables & beans every day so that your body gets the required energy along with all kinds of vitamins, minerals and fiber from the food items being consumed.

6 pm – 7 pm Evening Meal/Dinner (OPTION-2):
Chicken, Brown Rice & Veggies

Table 1.15 Recipe of the evening meal/dinner (OPTION2).

Food Item	Amount
Chicken (skinless, boneless, 1 Cup)	1 Cup
Brown Rice (1/4 Cup Dry, 1 Cup Cooked)	1 Cup
Mushrooms (Diced, 1 Cup)	1 Cup
Cucumbers (Organic, Fresh, 1/2 Cup)	1/2 Cup
Tomato (Organic, Fresh, 3/4 Cup)	3/4 Cup
Sea Salt (Very Little)	Little
Cayenne Pepper (Organic, 1 tsp)	1 tsp
Lemon Juice (2 tsp) + Purified Water	1 Cup

● Fresh cucumbers and fresh tomatoes are added to the meal using the measuring cups.

Table 1.16 Calories & nutritional information of the evening meal/dinner (OPTION2).

Food Item	Weight (gm)	Calories	Protein (gm)	Fat (gm)	Carbo (gm)
Chicken (skinless, boneless)	100	182.14	32.86	5	0
Brown Rice (1/4 Cup Dry, 1 Cup Cooked)	45	150	3	1.5	35
Mushrooms (Diced, 1 Cup)	100	28.57	2.71	0.29	4.43
Cucumbers (Organic, Fresh, 1/2 Cup)	100	16	0.6	0.1	3.6
Tomato (Organic, Fresh, 3/4 Cup)	100	20	1	0.2	4.25
Sea Salt (Very Little)	2	0	0	0	0
Cayenne Pepper (Organic, 1 tsp)	2	0	0	0	0
Lemon Juice (2 tsp) + Purified Water	30	8	0.2	0	2.4
Total →	479	404.71	40.37	7.09	49.68
Calories calculated →		424.01	161.48	63.81	198.72
Percentage (%) →			38.08%	15.05%	46.87%

● All food items are weighed using an electronic balance on the first day only.
● All food items are prepared using the measuring cups from the second day onwards.
● Fat: 9 calories/gm; Protein: 4 calories/gm; Carbohydrates: 4 calories/gm.

PREPARATION: Make your own evening meal /dinner with whole foods (skinless and boneless chicken, brown rice, vegetables, fresh tomatoes, fresh cucumbers and spices). Be consistent and consume the same quantity of each item of the meal (approximately the same calories) every day with the help of the measuring cups. Change and eat a variety of vegetables every day so that your body gets the required energy along with all kinds of vitamins, minerals and fiber from the food items being consumed.

IN-BETWEEN MEAL SNACKS

Table 1.17 In-between meal snack-I: Fruits.
During a typical day, I mostly eat one organic apple and one organic banana.
Sometimes I eat green grapes after the treadmill exercise or whenever my blood sugar goes low.

Food Item	Weight (gm)	Calories	Protein (gm)	Fat (gm)	Carbo (gm)	Sugar (gm)
Organic Banana (medium-size)	130	110	1	0	30	20
Organic Apple (medium-size)	150	130	1	0	34	25
Green Grapes (Seedless), 1 Cup	170	104	1	0	27	23

Fat: 9 calories/gm; Protein: 4 calories/gm; Carbohydrates: 4 calories/gm

Table 1.18 In-between meal snack-II: Nuts.
During a typical day, I mostly eat a handful of walnuts and a handful of blanched almonds.

Food Item	Weight (gm)	Calories	Protein (gm)	Fat (gm)	Carbo (gm)	Sugar (gm)
Walnuts, Dry Roasted, Handful, 28 g	28	170	4.0	16.0	5.0	1.0
Almonds, Blanched, Handful, 28 g	28	162	6.2	14.1	5.8	1.3
Pumpkin Seeds, Handful, 28 g	28	125	5.32	5.32	15.12	0.28

Fat: 9 calories/gm; Protein: 4 calories/gm; Carbohydrates: 4 calories/gm

Table 1.19 In-between meal snack-III: Protein bars (low-sugar).
I eat one protein bar sometimes at 3 pm or sometimes at 8 pm (only one bar a day).

Food Item	Weight (gm)	Calories	Protein (gm)	Fat (gm)	Carbo (gm)	Sugar (gm)
Protein Bar (Fibre-1)	33	140	6	6	17	7
Roasted peanuts, cocoa, milk, soy, etc.						
Protein Bar (Nature Valley)	37	190	11	11	13	8
Peanut butter, almonds, glucose, cocoa, etc.						
.						
Protein Bar (Nature Valley)	35	190	7	13	14	7
Roasted peanuts & sunflower seeds						

Fat: 9 calories/gm; Protein: 4 calories/gm; Carbohydrates: 4 calories/gm

Table 1.20 In-between meal snack-IV: Thai vegetable spring rolls.
I eat the Thai Spring Rolls as a snack every Sunday at around 3 pm (once a week):

Food Item	Weight (gm)	Calories	Protein (gm)	Fat (gm)	Carbo (gm)	Sugar (gm)
Thai Vegetable Spring Rolls (2 Rolls)		150	4	2	32	0

Fat: 9 calories/gm; Protein: 4 calories/gm; Carbohydrates: 4 calories/gm

TOTAL CALORIES: WEIGHT-LOSS DIET (LEVEL-I)

Table 1.21 Total calories being consumed in a typical day.

Food Item	Weight (gm)	Calories	Protein (gm)	Fat (gm)	Carbo (gm)
Breakfast (Organic Coffee, 1/2 Pita Bread)	55.3	76	3.32	0.82	14.16
Pre-Workout Meal (Egg-White Omelet)	897	371	21.73	11.47	44.22
Post-Workout Meal (Option-1)	474	496	41.6	10.91	66.15
Rotisserie Chicken, Brown Rice & Vegetables					
Evening Meal / Dinner (Option-1)	399	264	24.8	6.96	21.65
Baked Fish & Veggies					
In-Between Meal Snacks					
Organic Banana (medium-size)	130	110	1	0	30
Organic Apple (medium-size)	150	130	1	0	34
Green Grapes (Seedless), 1 Cup	170	104	1	0	27
Walnuts, Dry Roasted, Handful, 28 g	28	170	4	16	5
Almonds, Blanched, Handful, 28 g	28	162	6.2	14.1	5.8
Protein Bar (Nature Valley)	37	190	11	11	13
Peanut butter, almonds, glucose, cocoa, etc.					
Total →		2073	115.65	71.26	260.98
Calories Calculated →		2148	462.6	641.34	1043.92
Percentage (%) →			22%	30%	49%

Approximate Calories Per Day Calculated
Total Calories Being Consumed in a Typical Day   = 2073 Kcal
Total Protein Being Consumed in a Typical Day   = 115.65 g
Total Fat Being Consumed in a Typical Day   = 71.26 g
Total Carbohydrate Being Consumed in a Typical Day = 260.98 g

PROTEIN REQUIREMENT: The USDA (United States Dept. of Agriculture) recommends that an average healthy adult should get 10% to 35% of his or her calories from protein, or 0.8 grams of protein per kilogram of ideal body weight.

Protein Requirement (grams) = 0.8 x Body Weight (Kg)   (1 Kg = 2.2222 lb)
My body weight was 86 Kg. Therefore my protein requirement = 0.8 x 86 = 68.8 g.
So I have been consuming more than the sufficient amount of protein.

MY WEIGHT-LOSS JOURNAL USING WEIGHT-LOSS DIET (Level-I)

Table 1.22 My weight-loss journal using weight-loss diet (Level-I).

Date	Waist	Weight	Weight	BMI	Assessment
Units	(Inches)	(Kg)	(Pounds)	(Kg/m^2)	
Normal Range	< 34"	< 70 Kg	< 156 lb	18.5 to 24.9	
07-Feb-2015	First Diagnosed with Moderate Sleep Apnea (Index=22 to 28 Events/hr)				
07-Feb-2015	44	86	191	30.5	Obese
BMI = Weight (Kg) / Height (m)^2 = 86 / 1.68^2 = 30.5 = Obese					
19-Feb-2015	Committed to Lose Weight; Started Weight-Loss Diet (Level-I)				
12-Mar-2015	Started Exercising Every Day in the Gym (60 to 80 minutes/day).				
17-Apr-2015	43	84	187	29.8	Overweight
01-May-2015	42	83	184	29.4	Overweight
23-May-2015	42	84	187	29.8	Overweight
03-Jul-2015	41	82	182	29.1	Overweight
11-Jul-2015	40	80.5	179	28.5	Overweight
31-Jul-2015	39	80	178	28.3	Overweight
03-Aug-2015	39	79	176	28.0	Overweight
20-Aug-2015	39	80	178	28.3	Overweight
31-Aug-2015	39	80	178	28.3	Overweight
In 7 months, I lost only 6 Kg (13 Pounds); My weight loss was slow!					
My weight reached plateau; My sleep apnea is preventing my weight loss.					
08-Sep-2015	39	79	176	28.0	Overweight
06-Oct-2015	38	78.5	174	27.8	Overweight
11-Oct-2015	38	78.5	174	27.8	Overweight
10-Nov-2015	38	78.5	174	27.8	Overweight
25-Dec-2015	37	78	173	27.6	Overweight
28-Dec-2015	Oximetry Test Done: Desaturation Index = 6.9-8.4 Events/hr				
	I still have mild sleep apnea; However my weight reached plateau!				
14-Jan-2016	36.5	77	171	27.3	Overweight
19-Mar-2016	36	76.5	170	27.1	Overweight
19-Mar-2016	Oximetry Test Done: Desaturation Index = 4.6-4.8 Events/hr				
	I still have mild sleep apnea; However my weight reached plateau!				
27-May-2016	37	78	173	27.6	Overweight
12-Sep-2016	38.5	78	173	27.6	Overweight
My Weight Loss Was Very Slow; My Belly Fat and Weight Started Going Up.					
I Took Action; I Decided to Do Something About It and Researched.					
I Created Weight-Loss Diet (Level-II), Which Helped Me Loss Weight Fast.					

Table 1.23 Assessment guidelines for sleep apnea and weight loss.

Desaturation Index	Assessment		BMI (Kg/m^2)	Assessment
0 - 4 Events/hr	Normal (No Sleep Apnea)		< 18.5	Underweight
5 - 14 Events/hr	Mild Sleep Apnea		18.5 to 24.9	Normal
15 - 29 Events/hr	Moderate Sleep Apnea		25.0 to 29.9	Overweight
≥ 30 Events/hr	Severe Sleep Apnea		≥ 30	Obese

CONCLUSION
My Weight Loss Has Been Very Slow; My Belly Fat and Weight Started Going Up Again.

In 2004, I lost 35 Lb in 6 Weeks Just by Doing Treadmill, Without Watching Diet.
In 2006, I lost 35 Lb in 6 Weeks Just by Doing Treadmill, Without Watching Diet.
In 2008, I lost 35 Lb in 6 Weeks Just by Doing Treadmill, Without Watching Diet.
In 2011, I lost 35 Lb in 6 Weeks Just by Doing Treadmill, Without Watching Diet.

In 2015, I Tried to Do the Same But It Did Not Work.
I Figured Out the Reason: My Sleep Apnea Has Been Preventing My Weight Loss.

I Decided to Do Something About It and Researched; I Took Action.
I Created Weight-Loss Diet (Level-II), Which Helped Me Loss Weight Fast (see next page).

WEIGHT-LOSS DIET (LEVEL-II)
Daily Calories Intake: 1000 Calories
RAPID WEIGHT LOSS METHOD

INTRODUCTORY COMMENTS
Weight-Loss Diet (Level-I) = 2000 Kcal
Weight-Loss Diet (Level-II) = 1000 Kcal

When I tried the weight-loss diet (level-I) for 20 months, my weight dropped from 86 Kg (190 lb) to 78 Kg (175 lb), and I lost only 8 Kg or 18 pounds.

I needed to lose al least another 8 Kg or 18 pounds to attain normal body weight. I checked everything, and figured out the following flaws.

I Figured Out the Following Flaws While On the Weight-Loss Diet (Level-I):

1. MAJOR OBSTACLE: MY SLEEP APNEA HAD BEEN PREVENTING MY WEIGHT LOSS. Because I have sleep apnea, my brain mistakenly thinks that I would be starving in the near future and causes the liver to store and hold the fat for future use.

2. Also because I have sleep apnea, my SpO2 level (percentage saturation of oxygen in the blood) drops significantly and would not be normal throughout the day. So my resting metabolism slows down, resulting in the sluggish weight loss or no weight loss.

3. My metabolism most probably slowed down because of my age (as I was getting older). Also I was diagnosed with obstructive sleep apnea that kept my weight steady no matter how hard I tried to lose it.

4. My lower leg pain and my plantar fasciitis did not allow me to do high-intensity exercise. So I was not able to burn sufficient calories during exercise.

5. I didn't take my weight loss plan seriously and wasn't disciplined enough. I had been cheating on my diet, and had been eating junk foods in restaurants.

JUNK FOODS are strategically manufactured using processed foods and refined foods, adding large quantities of sugar, salt, oil, fat and several other chemicals including artificial colors and flavors that boost our cravings. So we tend to buy more and eat more of these foods. Junk foods sabotage our weight-loss efforts. I had been eating here and there, consuming pizza slices, chicken donair in the Middle-eastern Joints, pita bread, whole wheat bread, deep-fried samosas and spring rolls, Oh HENRY bars, chocolate chewy candies, dipped cone, ice cream, cashew clusters, Diet Coke, Diet Pepsi, excessive fruits, and other snacks every now and then, which was probably a major mistake.

So I decided to put a stop to consuming junk foods completely by exercising high willpower and high self-discipline. Healthy eating habits are essential to keep up with any weight-loss plan. This decision has helped me tremendously to quick-start my weight-loss plan, and the fat in my belly melted away quickly and easily.

I Took Action and Created the Weight-Loss Diet (Level-II)

1. I drastically reduced the daily calorie instate from 2000 Kcal to 1000 Kcal.

2. I drastically reduced the fat content to almost zero in my diet.
 When I don't consume fat, my body consumes my own fat (this is what happened).

3. I eliminated all animal products (the chicken and fish I had been eating before) from my diet plan as they contain high fat.

4. I exercised high willpower and high self-discipline. I wanted to lose weight & reverse my sleep apnea. I stopped eating all junk foods made from processed and refined foods in my diet and started eating whole foods only.

5. I minimized my salt and oil consumption (I was consuming too much salt and too much oil before).

6. I replaced all my in-between meal snacks with crunchy and tasty organic Kamut puffs.

7. I introduced unpasteurized and unfiltered organic apple cider vinegar with the mother to my diet, taking it 2 to 3 times a day with a straw, which probably contributed to some extent in my weight loss program.

8. I started drinking 16 cups of purified water per day compared to 8 cups per day.

9. I did not have hunger attacks, and had no cravings of any kind even though I drastically reduced my daily calorie intake and consumed only 1000 Kcal per day. My energy levels are normal.

10. When I created the Weight-Loss Diet (Level-II), my fat melted away quickly against all odds. I lost weight fast, and my body attained normal weight within 6 weeks. My body mass index (BMI) reached perfectly normal. More interestingly, my Obstructive Sleep Apnea (OSA) has disappeared.

8 am – 9 am Breakfast

Do not consume heavy breakfasts when resting at home.

Table 1.24 Recipe of the breakfast.

Food Item	Amount
Organic Coffee (10 g Brewed)	1 Cup
2% Organic Milk	2 tbsp
Kamut Puffs Organic	1 Cup

Table 1.25 Calories and nutritional information of the breakfast.

Food Item	Weight (gm)	Calories	Protein (gm)	Fat (gm)	Carbo (gm)
Organic Coffee (10 g Brewed to 1 Cup)	10	4	0.28	0.05	0
2% Organic Milk (2 tbsp)	15	7	0.54	0.27	0.66
Kamut Puffs Organic (1 Cup)	20	50	2	0	11
Total →	45	61	2.82	0.32	11.66
Calories calculated →		60.8	11.28	2.88	46.64
Percentage (%) →			19%	5%	77%

11 am - 12 pm Pre-Workout Meal: Egg-White Omelet with Veggies
It Could Be Your LUNCH / BRUNCH

Table 1.26 Recipe of the pre-workout meal (egg-white omelet with veggies). It is exactly the same recipe used in Weight-Loss Diet (Level-I).

Food Item/Ingredient	Amount
Egg White (extra large organic Eggs)	2
(98% of Egg Yolk is removed with a spoon)	
Broccoli (organic)	1 cup
Cauliflower (organic)	
(Replace this with Egg Plant/Other)	
Kale (organic)	1 cup
(Replace this with Spinach/Cilatro/Parsley/Other)	
Radishes (3 with stems)	3
(Replace this with your favorite vegetable)	
Bell Peppers (Red/Yellow/Green)	1/2 cup
Red Onion (organic)	1 cup
(Replace this with Yellow Onion)	
Ginger (fresh, peeled)	1/2 cup
Garlic (fresh, peeled, 4 cloves)	4 cloves
Sea Salt (a little bit)	a little
Curry Powder (organic)	1 tsp
Cayenne Pepper (organic)	1 tsp
Turmeric (organic root powder)	1/2 tbsp
Flaxseed (organic, ground)	1 spoon
Extra Virgin Olive Oil (a little)	A little
Purified Water (250 mL)	1 cup

11 am – 12 pm Pre-Workout Meal: Egg-White Omelet with Veggies
It is exactly the same recipe used in Weight-Loss Diet (Level-I).

Table 1.27 Calories & nutritional information of the pre-workout meal
(egg-white omelet with veggies).

Food Item	Weight	Calories	Protein	Fat	Carbo
	(gm)		(gm)	(gm)	(gm)
Egg White (2 Ex Large Organic Eggs)	94	50	10	0	0
(98% of Egg Yolk is removed with a spoon)					
Broccoli (Organic, 1 Cup)	80	26	2.5	0.30	4.7
Cauliflower (Organic, 1 Cup)	120	25	2.0	0	5.3
(Replace this with Egg Plant/Other)					
Kale (Organic, 1 Cup)	40	20	1.31	0.30	4
(Replace this with Spinach/Cilatro/Parsley/Other)					
Radishes (3 with stems)	60	10	0.42	0.06	2
(Replace this with your favorite vegetable)					
Bell Peppers (Red/Yellow/Green 1/2 Cup)	60	15	0.50	0	4
Red Onion (Organic, 1 Cup)	80	30	1	0.15	7
(Replace this with Yellow Onion)					
Ginger (Fresh, Peeled, 1/2 Cup)	60	30	0	0	6
Garlic (Fresh, Peeled, 4 cloves)	20	20	0	0	5.2
Sea Salt (a Little Bit)	2	0	0	0	0
Curry Powder (Organic, 1 tsp)	2	5	0	0	1
Cayenne Pepper (Organic, 1 tsp)	2	6	0	0	1
Turmeric (Organic Root Powder, 1/2 tbsp)	7	24	1	1	4
Flaxseed (Organic, Ground), 1 Spoon	15	70	3	5	0
Extra Virgin Olive Oil (A Little, 5 mL)	5	40	0	4.7	0
Purified Water (1 Cup=250 mL)	250	0	0	0	0
Total →	897	371	21.73	11.47	44.22
Calories calculated →		367.03	86.92	103.23	176.88
Percentage (%) →			23.68%	28.13%	48.19%

- All food items are weighed using an electronic balance on the first day only.
- All food items are prepared using the measuring cups from the second day onwards.
- Fat: 9 calories/gm; Protein: 4 calories/gm; Carbohydrates: 4 calories/gm.

See Figure 1.3 for a photograph of Egg-White omelet served on a plate.

HOW TO MAKE BOILED EGG WHITE & HOW TO PEEL THE SHELL
CHOOSE ORGANIC EXTRA LARGE RAW/WHOLE EGGS

In the Weight-Loss Diet (Level-II), I started consuming egg-white only for all my protein needs. All the protein comes from egg white only (no animal products).

● When I make the pre-workout meal "egg-white omelet with veggies," I discard the egg yolk, and add only the egg white to the vegetables and spices.

● When I make the post-workout meal and evening meal, I eat the boiled egg white. I boil the organic extra large whole egg, remove and discard the egg yolk, and consume the egg white only along with the boiled vegetables, beans and spices.

1. Always buy the fresh organic raw eggs, preferably extra large, after checking the expiration date, and make sure that there is a lot of time left before you consume. Before you cook and consume them, test them to know that they are not rotten. In order to test, leave the eggs in a large bowl of cold water. If the eggs sink and lay on their sides all the way down to the bottom of the bowl, that means they are good eggs and are not spoiled or rotten. If the eggs stand upright and float in the water, it means they are spoiled or rotten, and you should not eat them, just discard them. Do the same test before making the egg-white omelet every day.

2. Place the whole eggs gently in a medium saucepan filled with hot water, and boil them for 15 min on medium/high heat on the stove. Then leave the boiled eggs in cold water for a few minutes so that you can touch them, and then leave them in the fridge for several hours or overnight. It becomes easier to peel the eggshell if the boiled eggs are left in the fridge for several hours or overnight.

3. After the boiled egg was left in the fridge for several hours or overnight, remove the boiled egg from the fridge, break the shell all over the egg by beating on the shell with the unsharpened side of a knife (around the middle of the boiled egg, and around the front end and back end), but do not peel the egg shell yet. Leave this beaten egg in the boiled water on the stove again, and boil the beaten egg at medium or high heat for a few more minutes. Then take it out from the stove, leave it in a bowl of cold water for a few minutes, and then peel the shell. The shell comes off perfectly without losing any egg white. <u>Your goal is not to lose any amount of egg white</u>. Do not start peeling the shell immediately after boiling, if you do, you may not be able peel easily, and you may lose some egg white sticking to the eggshell.

4. After peeling the eggshell, cut the boiled egg at the center with a knife by making an incision of one inch long. Then open the egg white by pressing it with both hands, and you would see the solid yellowish ball of egg yolk without damage if the egg was boiled and cooled properly. You can either save this egg yolk for other family members or for your pets, or you can dump it in the garbage can. Now you have extracted 100% of the egg white from the egg without any loss.

5. After that, cut the boiled egg white into very small pieces (as small as possible) using a knife. Then add these small pieces of egg white to the boiled vegetables and boiled black beans so that protein (egg white is 100% protein) would be evenly distributed throughout the meal. Then you would have some tiny bit of protein with every bite of the meal you consume so that the digestion process would be optimized.

THIS IS WHAT I DO: I boil 6 organic extra large eggs at a time and leave them in the fridge. They last 3 days as I eat 2 boiled egg whites per day. When I take the boiled and cooled whole egg directly from the fridge, I beat it all over the egg (around the central part of the shell, around the front end and on the back end) with the unsharpened side of a knife and boil the egg under high heat for a few minutes. I then place the egg in cold water for a few seconds. The eggshell then peels off very easily without any loss of egg white. I then remove and discard egg yolk. <u>I then cut the egg white into very tiny pieces using a knife and mix them with semi-boiled vegetables and boiled black beans so that the protein is evenly distributed throughout the meal, and then I consume it.</u>
Always remember: Egg white is one 100% protein.

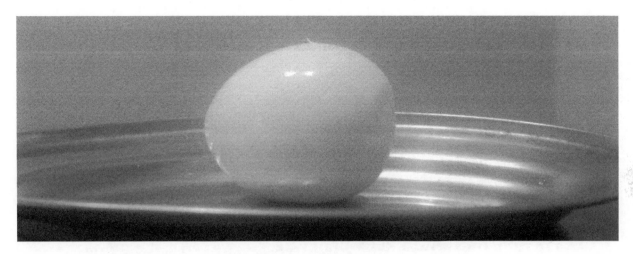

Figure 1.7 Extra large organic egg (boiled & peeled).

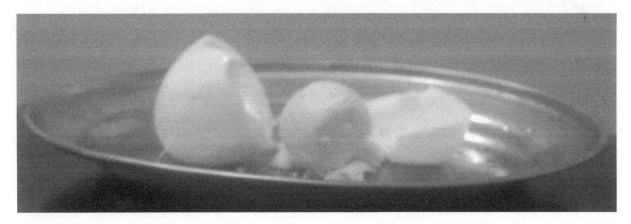

Figure 1.8 Extra large organic egg (boiled, peeled, cut in the middle & yolk removed).

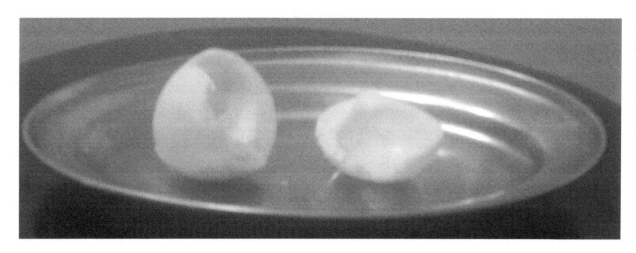

Figure 1.9 Extra large organic egg (boiled, peeled, cut in the middle, yolk removed & discarded).

This boiled egg white is cut into small pieces, mixed with boiled vegetables & consumed. Each extra large organic boiled egg white contains 5 g of protein. So consume as much boiled egg white as you wish until it meets your body's protein requirement. Always remember that egg white is one 100% protein. My goal was to eat high-protein and low-fat (or zero-fat) meals that helped me lose weight.

EAT MORE ORGANIC GREEN CABBAGE
Eat more semi-boiled organic green cabbage if you don't feel full. Cut the organic green cabbage into small pieces and semi-boil it for about 5 minutes in purified water. Add a pinch of sea salt and organic curry powder (no pepper needed). It is low in calories, very tasty and easily consumable with broth.

2 pm – 3 pm Post-Workout Meal
Cooked Vegetables & Boiled Egg White (Without Yolk)

Table 1.28 Recipe of the post-workout meal.

Food Item/Ingredients	Amount
Organic Yams Peeled (> 1/2 Cup)	> 1/2 Cup
Organic Fresh Carrots (> 1/2 Cup)	> 1/2 Cup
Organic Celery (< 1 Cup)	< 1 Cup
Organic Green Cabbage (1 Cup)	> Cup
Organic Black Beans Boiled (1/2 Cup)	1/2 Cup
Egg White Ex Lg (Organic, Boiled, No Yolk)	1 Egg
Sea Salt (Very Little)	Little
Cayenne Pepper (Organic, 1 tsp)	1 tsp
Purified Water (1 Cup)	1 Cup

● All fresh vegetables are washed, dried and cut into small pieces, and then measured using the measuring cups before cooking.

Table 1.29 Calories & nutritional information of the post-workout meal.

Food Item	Weight (gm)	Calories	Protein (gm)	Fat (gm)	Carbo (gm)
Organic Yams Peeled (> 1/2 Cup)	50	58	0.74	0.07	13.84
Organic Fresh Carrots (> 1/2 Cup)	50	17	0.37	0.06	3.9
Organic Celery (< 1 Cup)	70	11.2	0.49	0.14	2.1
Organic Green Cabbage (1 Cup)	90	26.8	1.28	0.128	6.4
Organic Black Beans Boiled (1/2 Cup)	85	112.1	7.51	0.44	20.2
Egg White Ex Lg (Organic, Boiled, No Yolk)	47	25	5	0	0
Sea Salt (Very Little)	2	0	0	0	0
Cayenne Pepper (Organic, 1 tsp)	2	0	0	0	0
Purified Water (1 Cup)	250	0	0	0	0
Total →	596	192.1	14.65	0.768	32.6
Calories calculated →		195.912	58.6	6.912	130.4
Percentage (%) →			29.91%	3.53%	66.56%

● All food items are weighed using an electronic balance on the first day only.
● All food items are prepared using the measuring cups from the second day onwards.
● Fat: 9 calories/gm; Protein: 4 calories/gm; Carbohydrates: 4 calories/gm

PREPARATION: Make your own post-workout meal with whole foods (cooked vegetables of your liking and boiled egg white without yolk and spices). Boiled egg white and boiled black beans are sources of protein. Be consistent and consume the same quantity of each item (approximately the same calories) every day with the help of the measuring cups. Change and eat a variety of vegetables every day so that your body gets the required energy along with all kinds of vitamins, minerals and fiber from the food items being consumed. Add more cooked green cabbage if you don't feel full.

6 pm – 7 pm   Evening Meal/Dinner
Cooked Vegetables & Boiled Egg White (Without Yolk)

Table 1.30 Recipe of the evening meal/dinner.

Food Item/Ingredients	Amount
Red Cabbage Crushed (1 Cup)	> 1 Cup
Boiled Fresh Carrots (> 1/2 Cup)	> 1/2 Cup
Cucumbers (Organic, fresh)	1/2 Cup
Tomato (medium-sized)	1
Egg White Ex Lg (Organic, Boiled, No Yolk)	1 Egg
Sea Salt (Very Little)	Little
Cayenne Pepper (Organic, 1 tsp)	1 tsp
Purified Water (1 Cup)	1 Cup

● Cucumbers and tomatoes are eaten fresh after measuring them using the measuring cups.

Table 1.31 Calories & nutritional information of the evening meal/dinner.

Food Item	Weight (gm)	Calories	Protein (gm)	Fat (gm)	Carbo (gm)
Red Cabbage Crushed (1 Cup)	140	40	2	0	8
Boiled Fresh Carrots (> 1/2 Cup)	50	17	0.37	0.06	3.9
Cucumbers (Organic, fresh)	100	16	0.6	0.1	3.6
Tomato (medium-sized)	150	30	1.5	0.3	6.5
Egg White Ex Lg (Organic, Boiled, No Yolk)	47	25	5	0	0
Sea Salt (Very Little)	2	0	0	0	0
Cayenne Pepper (Organic, 1 tsp)	2	0	0	0	0
Purified Water (1 Cup)	250	0	0	0	0
Total →	601	88	7.47	0.46	14
Calories calculated →		90.02	29.88	4.14	56
Percentage (%) →			33.19%	4.60%	62.21%

● All food items are weighed using an electronic balance on the first day only.
● All food items are prepared using the measuring cups from the second day onwards.
● Fat: 9 calories/gm; Protein: 4 calories/gm; Carbohydrates: 4 calories/gm

PREPARATION: Make your own evening meal with whole foods (cooked vegetables of your liking and boiled egg white without yolk and spices). Boiled egg white is a source of protein (you can add boiled black beans to this meal). Be consistent and consume the same quantity of each item of the meal (approximately the same calories) every day with the help of the measuring cups. Change and eat a variety of vegetables every day so that your body gets the required energy along with all kinds of vitamins, minerals and fiber from the food items being consumed. Add more cooked green cabbage if you don't feel full.

IN-BETWEEN MEAL SNACKS: ORGANIC KAMUT PUFFS

Table 1.32 Calories & nutritional information of organic kamut puffs.

Food Item	Weight (gm)	Calories	Protein (gm)	Fat (gm)	Carbo (gm)	Sugar (gm)
Kamut Puffs (organic, 1 cup)	20	50	2	0	11	0

In weight-loss diet (level-II), I replaced all the In-Between Meal Snacks with Kamut Puffs. Kamut is a brand name for an ancient heritage grain called khorasan wheat. The only ingredient in Kamut Puffs is whole wheat. Whenever I feel hungry in between two meals, I eat a cup of Organic Kamut Puffs. This habit I developed helped me lose weight.

ORGANIC KAMUT PUFFS is a healthy refreshment or snack with calories=50 calories per cup, dietary fiber=2 g per cup, protein=2 g per cup, sugar=0, total fat=0, sodium=0, GMO free, flavorful, crunchy, unbelievably tasty and refreshing.
In addition, I also eat 1 organic banana and 1 organic apple per day.

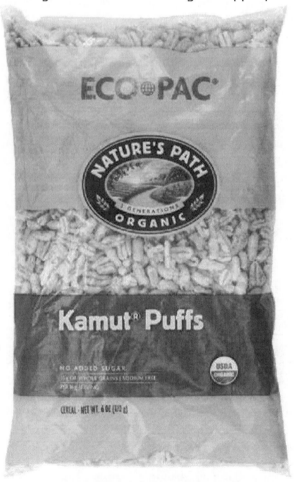

Courtesy of Nature's Path
Figure 1.10 The picture of a pack of organic kamut puffs.

TOTAL CALORIES: WEIGHT-LOSS DIET (LEVEL-II)

Table 1.33 Total calories being consumed in a typical day.

Food Item	Weight (gm)	Calories	Protein (gm)	Fat (gm)	Carbo (gm)
Breakfast (Organic Coffee, 1 Cup Kamut Puffs)	45	61	2.82	0.32	11.66
Pre-Workout Meal (Egg-White Omelet)	897	371	21.73	11.47	44.22
Post-Workout Meal	596	192.1	14.65	0.768	32.6
Veggies and Boiled Organic Egg White					
Evening Meal	601	88	7.47	0.46	14
Veggies and Boiled Organic Egg White					
In-Between Meal Snacks					
Organic Banana (medium-size)	130	110	1	0	30
Organic Apple (medium-size)	150	130	1	0	34
Kamut Puffs Organic, Nature's Path (1 Cup)	20	50	2	0	11
Kamut Puffs Organic, Nature's Path (1 Cup)	20	50	2	0	11
Total →		1052.1	52.67	13.02	188.48
Calories Calculated →		1082	210.68	117.162	753.92
Percentage (%) →			19%	11%	70%

Approximate Calories Per Day Calculated

Total Calories Being Consumed in a Typical Day = 1052 Kcal
Total Protein Being Consumed in a Typical Day   = 52.67 g
Total Fat Being Consumed in a Typical Day   = 13.02 g
Total Carbohydrate Being Consumed in a Typical Day = 188.48 g

PROTEIN REQUIREMENT: The USDA (United States Dept. of Agriculture) recommends that an average healthy adult should get 10% to 35% of his or her calories from protein, or 0.8 grams of protein per kilogram of ideal body weight.
Protein Requirement (grams) = 0.8 x Body Weight (Kg)   (1 Kg = 2.2222 lb)
My body weight at this time was 78 Kg; my protein requirement = 0.8 x 78 = 62.4 g.
So I need to increase my protein consumption. I did that by adding cottage cheese to my diet.

FAT CONTENT: The fat content has been reduced from 71.26 g (Level-I diet) to 13 g (Level-II diet). Most of that 13 g of fat was coming from extra virgin olive oil and flax seeds I have been adding to my egg-white omelet. This means, excluding extra virgin olive oil and flax seeds, my Level-II diet would become a ZERO-FAT DIET. When I started the Level-II diet, my fat melted away day by day right in front of my eyes and my weight and my body mass index (BMI) dropped to perfectly normal quickly as shown in the table below. When I did not consume fat, my body consumed my own fat, resulting in rapid weight loss.

WEIGHT-LOSS AND SLEEP APNEA JOURNAL OF Dr. RK
Using Weight-Loss Diet Level-II (1000 Calories)

I started eating at home all items made from whole foods. I carefully eliminated all processed foods and refined foods I had been consuming. When I did that, I drastically reduced my daily calorie intake from 2000 Kcal to 1000 Kcal, my belly fat melted away day by day, right in front of my eyes, and my weight and my body mass index reached normal as shown in the table below. The Following Information is "The Proof That Obstructive Sleep Apnea Can Be Reversed By Losing Weight!"

Table 1.34 My weight-loss journal using weight-loss diet (Level-II).

Date	Waist	Weight	Weight	BMI	Assessment
Units	(Inches)	(Kg)	(Pounds)	(Kg/m^2)	
Normal Range	< 34"	< 70 Kg	< 156 lb	18.5 to 24.9	
14-Sep-2016	Started Weight-Loss Diet (Level-II); 1000 Calories/Day.				
	Started Doing Treadmill & Bike Every Day (60 to 90 min per day).				
14-Sep-2016	38.5	78	173	27.6	Overweight
BMI = Weight (Kg) / Height (m)^2 = 78 / 1.68^2 = 27.6 = Overweight					
15-Sep-2016	37	77	171	27.3	Overweight
18-Sep-2016	37	76	169	26.9	Overweight
19-Sep-2016	36	75	167	26.6	Overweight
27-Sep-2016	36	74	164	26.2	Overweight
02-Oct-2016	35.5	73.5	163	26.0	Overweight
02-Oct-2016	35.5	73.5	163	26.0	Overweight
02-Oct-2016	35.5	73.5	163	26.0	Overweight
04-Oct-2016	35	73	162	25.9	Overweight
11-Oct-2016	34	72	160	25.5	Overweight
18-Oct-2016	34	71	158	25.2	Overweight
27-Oct-2016	34	70	156	24.8	Normal
09-Nov-2016	33	69	153	24.4	Normal
18-Nov-2015	Oximetry Test Done: Desaturation Index = 1.2-1.3 Events/hr)				
22-Nov-2016	33	68.5	152	24.3	Normal
23-Nov-2016	32.5	68	151	24.1	Normal
29-Nov-2015	Oximetry Test Done: Desaturation Index = 0.6 Events/hr.				
When my body resumed normal weight, my sleep apnea disappeared.					
01-Dec-2016	32.5	68	151	24.1	Normal
08-Dec-2016	32.5	67.5	150	23.9	Normal
01-Jan-2017	33	68	151	24.1	Normal
05-Jan-2017	32	67	149	23.7	Normal
11-Jan-2017	32	67	149	23.7	Normal

My weight before I started my weight-loss diet (level-I) = 86 Kg = 190 lb
My current weight = 68 Kg = 150 lb (which is perfectly normal).

WHICH MEANS I LOST ALTOGETHER 40 lb and 12 inches around my waist.
WHEN MY BODY RESUMED NORMAL WEIGHT, MY SLEEP APNEA DISAPPEARED.
AND MY OVERALL HEALTH IMPROVED SIGNIFICANTLY.

MY GOAL WAS TO REVERSE SLEEP APNEA BY LOSING WEIGHT.
I HAVE ACCOMPLISHED IT AND I NO LONGER SLEEP WITH CPAP THE MACHINE.

For the complete details about Reversing Sleep Apnea course, refer to the separate eBook entitled REVERSING SLEEP APNEA (Proof that Sleep Apnea Can Be Reversed by Losing Weight) by Dr. RK who reversed his obstructive sleep apnea by losing weight.

http://reversingsleepapnea.com/

KEEPING MY WEIGHT AT 150 lb IS NOW A CHALLENGE. I AM NOW WORKING ON THAT AND I AM CONFIDENT THAT I WOULD MAINTAIN NORMAL WEIGHT FOR THE REST OF MY LIFE. AND MY SLEEP APNEA WOULD REMAIN REVERSED FOR THE REST OF MY LIFE.

IMPORTANT WEIGHT-LOSS TIPS

SECTION-I

1. LEARN THE IMPORTANCE OF WHOLE FOODS: Master the concept and learn how to recognize WHOLE FOODS, PROCESSED FOODS and REFINED FOODS. Develop the habit of eliminating PROCESSED FOODS and REFINED FOODS from your diet, either the full meal nor a snack. Keep that in mind whenever you go grocery shopping.

2. Learn How to Read Labels: When you shop for groceries, always look at the label for the list of ingredients, and if the label says it contains preservatives (mostly high sodium), artificial colors and flavors, saturated fat, trans fat, do not buy it.

3. Learn How to Count Calories: It is not that difficult to count calories. With a simple hand calculator (if you know how to do additions, subtractions and divisions), you can calculate the amount of carbohydrates, protein and fat in a meal of any kind. I am teaching that in this course (See Appendix-A). If you don't like calculations, you can still do it using measuring cups.

4. Stop Eating Out in Restaurants and Stop Buying Snacks, Sandwiches in Convenience Stores, Gas Stations & 7-Eleven. All those snacks are loaded with processed foods and refined foods. You would never find a meal made with whole foods in any restaurant. All the meals in all the restaurants are loaded with processed foods and refined foods, which inhibit weight loss and only add pounds to your belly. So if you are going to a restaurant means you are cheating on your diet. Even if you eat once a week in a restaurant, that would block your weight loss trend. Research and find out yourself (When I was losing weight with my diet, and ate buffet one day, my weight went up by 1 Kg by the next day).

5. Start Eating at Home: Cook your own meals with your favorite organic whole foods.

6. Eat Only Whole Foods, and Eliminate Processed Foods and Refined Foods from Your Meal: You can include whole chicken, whole fish and whole meat in the raw form (but not deep-fried, breaded or anything changed from its original form) in your diet along with boiled vegetables. But do not fry any item with a lot of oil. Instead, bake it or cook it with purified water, and after it is baked or cooked, sprinkle a few drops of extra virgin olive oil, sea salt, organic curry powder and organic cayenne pepper or other, and lemon juice so that it would be flavorful when you eat it. If you don't feel full with the quantity of the meal, then add more boiled organic green cabbage. Cut the organic green cabbage into small pieces before cooking, and boil it in purified water for about 5 minutes, and add sea salt and your favorite spice. Do not eat coleslaw dressed with tartar sauce or any kind of dressing.

7. Eat All Organic Foods: Organic eggs, organic vegetables, organic fruits, organic chicken, organic meat, salmon fish, sea salt or Kosher salt, organic spices, etc. Research proves that organic foods are more nutritious than conventional foods. Purchase fresh organic groceries once every week. Do not store organic foods for more than a week in your fridge, as they could lose nutritional values if you store them longer than a week.

IMPORTANT WEIGHT-LOSS TIPS

SECTION-II

8. Egg-White Omelet: It is the same meal (not changed) in Level-I diet or Level-II diet. Egg-White Omelet with Veggies keeps me alert all day long. It makes me feel full with a lot of energy to go to the gym and exercise for at least an hour. I have no hunger attacks or any kind of cravings during the day or in the night. It is the best meal of the day, and I simply enjoy this meal. I would eat this nutritious and delicious meal every day for the rest of my life.

9. Apple Cider Vinegar: I take 2 to 3 tablespoons of the unpasteurized and unfiltered BRAGG organic apple cider vinegar with mother 2 to 3 times a day just before meals in a glass of warm water, with a straw and a pinch of Cayenne pepper. It has been acting as a hunger suppressant and has been making my digestion process much easier. It has been contributing to lowering my blood-sugar levels as well.

10. In-Between Meal Snack "Kamut Puffs:" I eat 1 to 1.5 cups of Nature's Path Organic Kamut Puffs several times whenever I feel hungry in between meals. Kamut Puffs replaced all the high-calorie and high-fat snacks and junk foods, which have been blocking my weight loss. The crunchy and flavorful Organic Kamut Puffs became my favorite snack.

11. Organic Psyllium Husks: I take a large spoonful or 5 g of Organic Psyllium Husks, course powder, mixed with 1.5 cups of purified water every night before bedtime. It has been helping in my bowel movement. Discharging the stool every day on a continuous basis is of utmost importance in the weight loss program.

12. Purified Water: I drink 16 cups of purified water per day (including the water I use for cooking). The standard is 8 cups of water per day. I purchase purified water in Safeway where they produce and sell purified water by Reverse Osmosis, which removes chlorine, fluoride and other harmful chemicals & contaminants from tap water. This high water consumption has been helping in my digestion, flushing the melted and dissolved fat away through urination, and at the same time keeping my organs and other body parts lubricated, clean and healthy.

13. Organic Coffee: I drink 2 to 3 cups of organic coffee by adding 2 tbsp of 1% organic milk every day before going to the gym (before noon). The coffee gives me energy and keeps me alert throughout the day, and saves me from the afternoon sleepiness.

14. Multivitamins: I take multivitamins every day. When I am consuming low-calorie diet deliberately to lose weight, my body needs to be supplemented with multivitamins, vitamin C (>1000 mg) and other supplements.

15. Insomnia: I treated my INSOMNIA before treating my weight gain and sleep apnea. A good night's sleep is very important if you want to lose weight. Fix the INSOMNIA first.

16. HIGH WILLPOWER & HIGH SELF-DISCIPLINE are essential to lose weight.
In order to keep away from eating out at restaurants, and to eliminate processed foods and refined foods, which are classified as JUNK FOODS in your meal, you need to practice and possess high willpower and high self-discipline.

IF YOU WANT TO LOSE WEIGHT AND LIVE WELL, YOU SHOULD DEVELOP HEALTHY EATING HABITS!

>>>>>>>>THE END OF "REVERSING OBESITY" MAIN ARTICLE <<<<<<<<

CHAPTER 2   HOW TO COUNT CALORIES

TABLE OF CONTENTS

CONCEPT OF CALORIES [1, 2]

Energy offered by any food item is expressed in "calories." A calorie is the unit of heat in the international system (SI) of units. Heat is the kinetic energy transfer from one medium to another. A calorie is defined as the amount of energy transfer required to raise the temperature of one cubic centimeter of pure water (provided the water temperature is above the freezing point and below the boiling point) by one degree centigrade. Water is said to be pure if its density is perfectly 1 gm/cm^3. All foods have calories. A calorie is a small unit.

Food scientists refer to and count food calories in "Kilocalories." One Kilocalorie is equivalent to 1000 calories. For example, one tablespoon of granulated sugar weighing 12 grams has 46 Kcal. That means 12 grams of granulated sugar offers 46 Kilocalories of energy. In calorie counter tables, it is usually listed as "46 cal" instead of 46 Kcal. "Calories or Cal" is a slang word being used in the food industry to represent Kcal. So the confusion between calories and kilocalories has to be clarified. In some other books, food calories are expressed in Kilojoules (KJ).
1 KJ = 0.238 Kcal or 1 Kcal = 4.2 KJ.

So the actual definition is: "One Kilocalorie (Kcal) is the amount of heat necessary to raise the temperature of one kilogram of water by one degree centigrade."

The energy content of a food item can be determined by means of a bomb calorimeter. A food sample of known weight is burned in an atmosphere of pure oxygen in a jacketed bomb calorimeter. The heat released by the burned food is absorbed by the water in the jacket. The amount of energy is then calculated from the rise in water temperature and the weight of the food sample. There are several scientific methods developed and being used by food scientists to experimentally determine the nutritional composition (protein, fat and carbohydrate content) of any food item.

Table 2.1 Standard food calories of nutrients.

All food items that humans consume comprise carbohydrates, fats and proteins. After thorough research, food scientists have established the following facts:
• Carbohydrates have approximately 4 Calories Per Gram.   • Fat has approximately 9 Calories Per Gram.   • Protein has approximately 4 Calories per Gram.   • Alcohol has approximately 7 Calories Per Gram.

EXAMPLE CALCULATION-I

How to Calculate the Calories (Energy) Offered by a Food Item
By knowing the amounts of carbohydrates, fats and proteins present in a food item, it is possible to calculate the total calories or the energy being offered by that food item. For example, Avalon Dairy posted the nutritional information for 2% organic milk as follows (see the label shown below).

Table 2.2 Avalon Label: Calories and nutritional information of 2% organic milk. [3]

```
┌─────────────────────────────────────────┐
│ Nutrition Facts                          │
│ Valeur nutritive                         │
│ Per 1 cup (250 mL) / par 1 tasse (250 mL)│
│ Amount                      % Daily Value │
│ Teneur                 % valeur quotidienne│
├─────────────────────────────────────────┤
│ Calories / Calories 130                  │
│ Fat / Lipides 5 g                    8 %  │
│   Saturated / saturés 3 g                 │
│   + Trans / trans 0.2 g             17 %  │
│ Cholesterol / Cholestérol 20 mg      7 %  │
│ Sodium / Sodium 130 mg               5 %  │
│ Carbohydrate / Glucides 12 g         4 %  │
│   Fibre / Fibres 0 g                 0 %  │
│   Sugars / Sucres 12 g                    │
│ Protein / Protéines 9 g                   │
│ Vitamin A / Vitamine A              15 %  │
│ Vitamin C / Vitamine C               6 %  │
│ Calcium / Calcium                   30 %  │
│ Iron / Fer                           0 %  │
│ Vitamin D / Vitamine D              45 %  │
└─────────────────────────────────────────┘
```

3. Avalon Dairy 2% Organic Milk (Nutritional Information)
http://www.avalondairy.com/organic-milk/

I have tabulated the values of calories, carbohydrates, fats and proteins of the Avalon label in the table below:

Table 2.3 Calories and nutritional information of 2% organic milk.

Food Item	Weight	Calories	Protein	Fat	Carbo
	(gm)		(gm)	(gm)	(gm)
Avalon Dairy 2% Orgaic Milk (1 cup)	250	130	9.0	5.0	12.0

Calories are calculated as follows:
1 cup of 2% organic milk has 12 g of carbohydrates. Therefore 12 x 4 = 48 calories
1 cup of 2% organic milk has 5 g of fats.   Therefore 5 x 9 = 45 calories
1 cup of 2% organic milk has 9 g of proteins.   Therefore 9 x 4 = 36 calories

Therefore 1 Cup of 2% organic milk offers 48 + 45 + 36 = 129 calories of energy.
Avalon Dairy already posted on the label that 1 cup of 2% organic milk has 130 calories. So the 129 calories that I just calculated matched with 130 calories posted.

Which means if you know the amounts of carbohydrates, fats and proteins present in a food item, you can calculate the total calories being offered by that food item.
++

EXAMPLE CALCULATION-II
HOW TO CALCULATE THE CALORIES OF A MEAL ON A DINNER PLATE DISTRIBUTION OF FAT, PROTEIN AND CARBOHYDRATES

Suppose you recently purchased the oven-baked Rotisserie chicken at Save-On-Foods supermarket, brought it home and dished out a handful of chicken breast from the whole chicken, and placed it on your dinner plate. You also placed 1.5 cups of cooked brown rice, and 1/2 cup of cooked/boiled black beans on your dinner plate along with a pinch of sea salt & Cayenne pepper. So your dinner plate has 3 food items: Rotisserie chicken breast, cooked brown rice and boiled black beans. You want to calculate the total calories and the distribution of fat, protein and carbohydrates in your meal.

THIS IS WHAT YOU SHOULD DO
1. Determine the weight of each food item on your dinner plate using an electronic balance. For example,
a. Rotisserie Chicken Breast On Your Dinner Plate   = 125 g
b. Cooked Brown Rice (1.5 Cups) On Your Dinner Plate = 67.5 g
c. Cooked Black Beans (1/2 Cup) On Your Dinner Plate   = 85 g

2. Find out the standard nutritional information (calories, fat, protein & carbohydrates) for Rotisserie chicken, cooked brown rice and cooked black beans.
You can find this nutritional information:
a. On the label of the package (with food item) you purchased.
b. In the handbooks of nutritional values/calorie-counting tables
c. By doing a Google search on the internet

By doing a Google search, I found the following values (calories, protein, fat and carbohydrates) for Rotisserie chicken, cooked brown rice and cooked black beans.

Table 2.4 Calories and nutritional information of Rotisserie ckicken meal from Google search.

Food Item	Weight	Calories	Protein	Fat	Carbo
	(gm)		(gm)	(gm)	(gm)
Rotisserie Chicken Breast(1 Cup)	100	148	29	4.00	0
Brown Rice (1/4 Cup Dry, 1 Cup Cooked)	45	150	3	1.5	35
Organic Cooked Black Beans (1 Cup)	172	227	15.2	0.9	40.8

I got the following URLs when I did the Google search:

Google search: calories Rotisserie chicken breast
http://www.myfitnesspal.com/food/calories/kds-rotisserie-chicken-breast-no-skin-387187970

Google search: calories cooked brown rice (short grain)
http://www.lundberg.com/product/organic-brown-short-grain-rice/

Google search: calories cooked black beans
https://draxe.com/black-beans-nutrition/
http://www.calorieking.com/foods/calories-in-fresh-or-dried-legumes-beans-black-boiled_f-ZmlkPTEzMDYwNg.html

3. Now that you know the nutritional breakdown (Protein, Fat & Carbohydrate content) for a given "Serving Size," you can calculate the same for any serving size or for any amount of food item or items on your dinner plate. The calculations are shown below:

Rotisserie Chicken:
For the Serving Size = 100 g, Calories = 148, Protein = 29 g, Fat = 4 g, Carbo = 0 g
For the Dinner Plate Size = 125 g, Calories = (125/100)(148) = 185 g
$$\text{Protein} = (125/100)(29) = 36.25 \text{ g}$$
$$\text{Fat} = (125/100)(4) = 5.0 \text{ g}$$
$$\text{Carbohydrates} = (125/100)(0) = 0 \text{ g}$$

Cooked Brown Rice
For the Serving Size = 45 g, Calories = 150, Protein = 3 g, Fat = 1.5 g, Carbo = 35 g
For the Dinner Plate Size = 67.5 g, Calories = (67.5/45)(150) = 225 g
$$\text{Protein} = (67.5/45)(3) = 4.5 \text{ g}$$
$$\text{Fat} = (67.5/45)(1.5) = 2.25 \text{ g}$$
$$\text{Carbohydrates} = (67.5/45)(35) = 52.5 \text{ g}$$

Cooked Black Beans
For the Serving Size = 172 g, Calories = 227, Protein = 15.2 g, Fat = 0.9 g, Carbo = 40.8 g
For the Dinner Plate Size = 85 g,   Calories = (85/172)(227) = 112.1 g
$$\text{Protein} = (85/172)(15.2) = 7.51 \text{ g}$$
$$\text{Fat} = (85/172)(0.9) = 0.44 \text{ g}$$
$$\text{Carbohydrates} = (85/172)(40.8) = 20.2 \text{ g}$$

4. After calculating the nutritional information for all food items on your dinner plate, arrange the values in a table as shown below, and then calculate the percentage distribution of protein, fat and carbohydrates in your meal.

Table 2.5 Calculations for the nutritional information of Rotisserie chicken meal.

Food Item	Weight	Calories	Protein	Fat	Carbo
	(gm)		(gm)	(gm)	(gm)
Rotisserie Chicken Breast(1 Cup)	125	185	36.25	5.00	0
Brown Rice (1.5 Cups Cooked)	67.5	225	4.5	2.25	52.5
Organic Black Beans Boiled (1/2 Cup)	85	112.1	7.51	0.44	20.2
Total →	277.5	522.1	48.26	7.69	72.7
Calories calculated →		553.05	193.04	69.21	290.8
Percentage (%) →			35%	13%	53%

- Protein has approximately 4 Calories per Gram.
- Fat has approximately 9 Calories Per Gram.
- Carbohydrates have approximately 4 Calories Per Gram.
- Alcohol has approximately 7 Calories Per Gram.

Protein Calories   = 48.26 x 4 = 193.04 calories
Fat Calories   = 7.69 x 9 = 69.21 calories
Carbohydrate Calories =72.7 x 4 = 290.80 calories
% Protein   = 193.0/(193 + 69.21 + 290.8) ≈ 35%
% Fat   = 69.21/(193 + 69.21 + 290.8) ≈ 12%
% Carbohydrates = 290.8/(193 + 69.21 + 290.8) ≈ 53%
TOTAL ≈ 100%

As shown above, you can do your own calculations using a simple hand calculator, and arrange all values in a table manually. Or you can use the Microsoft EXCEL program, and by means of simple formulae (for addition, multiplication and division) do the calculations. By copying and pasting the formulae from one cell to another, you can do the same kind of calculations for any kind of meal.

WHEN YOU CREATE A NEW DIET: You don't put whatever amounts of food items you want in the dinner plate (bowl) and do calorie counting as explained in the aforementioned example. Instead, you place the pre-determined amounts of food items (1 cup, 1/2 cup, 1/4 cup, etc.) and then take their weights using an electronic balance, only on the first day. From second day onwards, you create the same or a similar meal of which you have already done the calorie counting using measuring cups (1 cup, 1/2 cup, 1/4 cup, etc.). You don't have to weigh the items every day. You don't have to do calorie counting every day.

After you have extensive experience, you don't even need the measuring cups. You would be able guess the amount of any food item by simply placing a handful of the food item. So take a handful of that food item (approximately) in a bowl, and cook the whole meal. IT IS AS EASY AS COOKING REGULAR MEALS WITHOUT CALORIE COUNTING!

NUTRITIONAL INFORMATION OF LIQUID EGG WHITES

The following nutritional information for liquid egg whites is posted by Rabbit River Farms.

4. Calories and Nutritional Information of Liquid Egg Whites, Posted by Rabbit River Farms, Richmond, BC, Canada.
http://www.rabbitriverfarms.com/products/organic-eggs-2/

Table 2.6 Calories and nutritional information of liquid egg whites.

Food Item	Weight (gm)	Calories	Protein (gm)	Fat (gm)	Carbo (gm)
Egg Whites (1/2 cup)	47	25	5	0	0

Table 2.7 Label for the calories and nutritional information of liquid egg whites. [4]

Nutrient	amt	%dv
Liquid Egg Whites per 3 tbsp (47g)		
Calories	25	
Fat	0g	0%
Saturated Fat + Trans Fat	0g +0g	0%
Cholesterol	0mg	
Sodium	80mg	3%
Carbohydrate	0g	0%
Fibre	0g	0%
Sugars	0g	
Protein	5g	
Vitamin A		0%
Vitamin C		0%
Calcium		0%
Iron		0%

Extra Large Organic Eggs (Rabbit River Farms): I purchased this item in a Whole Foods store. I cracked one extra large whole organic egg in a small metal bowl, and removed 98% to 99% of egg yolk with a large spoon, and then weighed the egg white using an electronic balance.

I found that the weight of the egg white is approximately 47 g, matching the information on the label. Therefore I confirmed the following nutritional information for egg whites.

Table 2.8 Calculations for the calories and nutritional information of liquid egg whites.

Food Item	Weight (gm)	Calories	Protein (gm)	Fat (gm)	Carbo (gm)
Egg White (1 Ex Large Organic Eggs)	47	25	5	0	0
(98% of Egg Yolk is removed with a spoon)					
Egg White (2 Ex Large Organic Eggs)	94	50	10	0	0
(98% of Egg Yolk is removed with a spoon)					

ACCURATE CARBOHYDRATE COUNTING [1, 5, 6, 7, 8, 9]

The American Diabetes Association, some organizations related to nutrition and diabetes education, dietitians and weight loss experts recommended the following formula, making an effort to further correct the amount of total carbohydrates being printed on food labels:

Amount of Total Carbohydrates Corrected =
Total Carbohydrates (g) on the Label − Dietary Fiber (g) on the Label − 1/2 Sugar Alcohol (g) on the Label

The food manufacturers in some countries are required by law to publish a label on the manufactured item by revealing the total carbohydrates in grams. This total carbohydrates includes the amount of starch, dietary fiber, sugar and sugar alcohol. However dietary fiber does not raise blood-glucose levels. So it does not contribute to the energy content. Therefore the dietary fiber content in grams is to be entirely subtracted from total carbohydrates in grams in order to correct it. Sugar alcohol is a type of reduced-calorie sweetener, such as sorbitol, xylitol, mannitol, etc., added to food items by food manufacturers. But the research showed that sugar alcohols are only half-effective in raising blood-glucose levels. So only half of the sugar alcohol content in grams is to be subtracted from the total carbohydrates in grams in order to correct it.

IT IS IMPORTANT TO NOTE THAT WHOLE FOODS DO NOT CONTAIN SUGAR AND ALCOHOL BUT CONTAIN DIETARY FIBER AND SOME WHOLE FOODS MAY CONTAIN SUGAR. PROCESSED FOODS DO CONTAIN SUGAR ALCOHOL. If you eat only a whole food meal, you don't need to worry about sugar alcohol. Therefore the general rule is that the fiber content in grams and half of the sugar alcohol content in grams are to be subtracted from the total carbohydrates in grams listed on the label to obtain the accurate amount of carbohydrates that indeed represents the energy and contributes to raising blood-glucose levels. The amount of total carbohydrates corrected is to be multiplied by 4 to obtain the calories being offered by the total carbohydrates corrected.

IS CARBOHYDRATE CORRECTION NECESSARY?
IS THE DEDUCTION OF FIBER FROM CARBOHYDRATE NECESSARY?

I decided not to correct the amount of total carbohydrates being printed on the food labels while calculating calories in my weight-loss diet recipes because of the following reasons:

a. There are two types of dietary fiber: (i) soluble fiber that dissolves in water and is fermented in the colon to produce byproducts and (ii) insoluble fiber that does not dissolve in water and acts like a bulking agent mixed with water in order to sweep the wastes through the colon along with it. Insoluble fiber does not offer any energy so it has no calories. But soluble fiber does offer energy and therefore has calories. Food scientists have conducted research on soluble fiber and reported that the bacteria in the gut reacts with the water-soluble fiber, resulting in the production of short chain fatty acids, which offer some sort of energy.

Some dietitians have reported that soluble fiber offers 1.9 calories per gram. [7, 8] FDA reported that the amount of caloric contribution due to bacterial degradation is about 1.5 calories per gram of fiber. [6] So we cannot ignore the fact that soluble fiber has calories. As the food labels do not reveal how much soluble fiber is there in any food item, there is no way we can correct the amount of carbohydrates based on the fiber content.

Dr. Mike Roussell Wrote the Following: [10] Don't worry about improving the accuracy of your calorie-counting by being technically correct about the contribution of fiber. It is simply a wasted effort. If there is a caloric difference due to fiber, it's small enough that it's probably easily obliterated if you walk to work or take your dog for a stroll after dinner.

b. If you go by "accuracy," the counting of calories itself is only by approximation and there is no need to worry about the accuracy of the amount of carbohydrates.

As a matter of fact, when counting calories, all the aforementioned educators multiply the amount of carbohydrates by 4 instead of 4.1 or 4.2. If they want to count calories accurately, they should actually multiply the amount of carbohydrate in grams by 4.1 or 4.2 (not by 4). So there was an error generated already by multiplying by 4. Carbohydrates actually offer 4.1 or 4.2 calories per gram (4 calories per gram is an approximation or rounded value). Similarly fat has 9.5 calories per gram (not 9 calories per gram), and protein has 4.1 calories per gram (not 4 calories per gram). Different studies report different calories per gram of carbohydrates, fats and proteins. For example, in the article of Nutrition [11], it was reported that Carbohydrates have 4.2 Calories per gram, Fat has 9.5 Calories per gram and Protein has 4.1 Calories per gram.

And also Sadava, David and Orians, Gordon H. Life [12] reported the following values: Carbohydrates have 4.2 Calories per gram, Fat has 9.5 Calories per gram and Protein has 4.1 Calories per gram.

There was no general consensus reached regarding the energy values being offered by carbohydrates, fats and proteins. All calorie-counting calculations are by approximation as they are not the accurate values. So don't worry about accuracy.

c. More than that, when you deduct the amount of dietary fiber from the total carbohydrates and multiply by 4, your total daily calorie intake is going to be lower than that without deduction, which could trick your brain to feel free to eat more because your total calorie intake was lower. As a result, you could gain weight by eating more. If you do not deduct the dietary fiber from total carbohydrates, then you feel satisfied by the total daily calorie instate, and then you could lose weight by eating less.

d. In some countries, the food manufacturers don't even list the amount of dietary fiber so you never know how much fiber is to be deducted from the total carbohydrates. So the deduction of dietary fiber from the total carbohydrates is not universally verified and validated when counting calories.

e. Calorie counting should be used to compare the total daily calorie intake from one day to another. It is the relative calorie counting that is important, not the absolute calorie counting. From the approximate calorie count, you can either lower the total daily calorie intake by eating less or increase it by eating more. The approximate calorie counting, without worrying too much about its accuracy, should be used by keeping in mind that you should eventually eat less in an attempt to lose weight. That can be accomplished by means of the measuring cups, by using the 3/4 cup instead of the 1 cup or by using the 1 cup instead of the 1.5 cup, etc. on your dinner plate. By counting the number of cups you have been eating until today, you can easily lower the amount of food being consumed right from the next day, thereby accomplishing your weight loss goal. Healthy eating habits "such as eating whole foods" would allow you to consume lower calories, and lose weight. Accurate calorie counting is not going to help you lose weight. So don't worry too much about it!

CONCLUSION: The deduction of fiber from carbohydrate is unnecessary while counting calories of a food item or a meal. Approximate calorie-counting would do the job.

REFERENCES

1. Permanent Diabetes Control, Authored by Rao Konduru, MS, PhD, Reviewed by Dr. Marshall Dahl, MD, PhD.

2. Website www.mydiabetescontrol.com about Permanent Diabetes Control.

3. Avalon Dairy 2% Organic Milk (Nutritional Information)
http://www.avalondairy.com/organic-milk/

4. Calories and Nutritional Information of Liquid Egg Whites, Posted by Rabbit River Farms, Richmond, BC, Canada.
http://www.rabbitriverfarms.com/products/organic-eggs-2/

5. Demystifying Sugar: Diabetes Education Online, University of California, San Francisco, CA, USA.
https://dtc.ucsf.edu/living-with-diabetes/diet-and-nutrition/understanding-carbohydrates/demystifying-sugar/

6. Counting Carbohydrates like a Pro by Gary Scheiner, MS, CDE.
https://www.diabetesselfmanagement.com/nutrition-exercise/meal-planning/counting-carbohydrates-like-a-pro/

7. How to Correctly Count Calories? By Kelly M (with 57 Comments).
http://www.foodiefiasco.com/how-to-correctly-count-calories/

8. Dietary Fiber (Read Section: Fiber & Calories).
https://en.wikipedia.org/wiki/Dietary_fiber#Fiber_and_calories

9. Is a Calorie a Calorie? By Andrea C Buchholz and Dale A Schoeller, The American Journal of Clinical Nutrition.
http://ajcn.nutrition.org/content/79/5/899S.long#ref-28

10. Ask the Micromanager: Does Fiber Count in Calories? By Mike Roussell, PhD.
http://www.bodybuilding.com/fun/ask-the-macro-manager-does-fiber-count-in-calories.html

11. Nutrition.
https://www.brianmac.co.uk/nutrit.htm

The approximate energy yield per gram is as follows:
Carbohydrates = 4.2 Calories, Fat = 9.5 Calories and Protein = 4.1 Calories

12. Energy Density of Carbohydrates.
http://hypertextbook.com/facts/2007/AnuragPanda.shtml

CHAPTER 3: EAT WHOLE FOODS ONLY
Avoid Processed Foods and Refined Foods

TABLE OF CONTENTS

EAT WHOLE FOODS ONLY
Avoid Processed Foods and Refined Foods

WHOLE FOODS [1, 2, 3]

Whole foods are natural raw foods possessing all the nutrients nature bestowed upon them when they were grown and produced in orchards, gardens, or greenhouses. Whole foods are foods that have not been processed, modified or refined by any means by adding preservatives, colors and/or other additives in order to improve their taste and/or to store them for extended periods for the future consumption.

Whole foods are the healthiest foods for the human body. They are authentically flavorful, have vibrant colors and rich textures. Whole foods are loaded with carbohydrates, proteins, micronutrient vitamins, minerals, antioxidants, phytonutrients, fiber, and do not contain unhealthy fats.

Examples of Whole Foods

All raw foods, unprocessed, unrefined and unpolished whole grains, coarse grains (cracked, not powdered), beans, peas, vegetables, legumes, fruits, all unprocessed animal products (still in their whole form without any modification) such as whole chicken, whole turkey, whole beef, whole fish, whole eggs and all dairy products in their original form. Rotisserie chicken falls under the whole foods category but Kentucky Fried Chicken or any kind of deep-fried and breaded chicken is considered as processed food. See a complete list of "vegetables and greens" at the end of this chapter.

PROCESSED FOODS [3, 4, 5, 6, 7]

Processed foods are foods manufactured from whole foods or foods in a food factory, by adding preservatives, artificial colors and flavors including salt (sodium), MSG (monosodium glutamate), hydrogenated oils, fillers, sugars and sweeteners in order to package, transport and preserve them for sale in supermarkets.

Being modified, processed foods lose the nutritional value that the whole foods originally possessed. They also get contaminated with artificial colors, flavors and other additives making them harmful and unhealthy if consumed with ignorance.

Processed meats are manufactured in meat factories by adding a coloring agent called "sodium nitrite" to make them look fresh and attractive to consumers. Some processed meats contain monosodium glutamate (MSG), an even more harmful agent. People with unhealthy lifestyle habits choose processed meats, and they all pay a big price down the road. Research suggests that processed meats are directly linked to chronic health diseases and even cancer.

Processed meat contains several chemical compounds that are not naturally present in fresh meat. Many of these chemical compounds are harmful to health. All processed foods are "JUNK FOODS" with added taste so that people crave more of it. Junk Foods are made by adding loads of salt, sugar, a variety of fats, colors and flavors.

Junk foods taste good tricking your brain to want more and more. Processed foods are harder to digest and make people fat and cause diseases. Processed Meats are too dangerous for human consumption. World Cancer Research International established that there is a link between processed foods and cancer.

Examples of Processed Foods

● Processed meat, red meat, processed pork, all meats that have been smoked, salted, cured, dried and canned, corned beef, beef jerky, bacon, ham, meat loaf, hot dogs, frozen pizza with processed meat, kid's meal containing red meat, ravioli and meat pasta foods, meat balls with spaghetti, fried chicken, breaded chicken, fish and beef, salami, pepperoni, sausages (chicken, turkey, beef), sausage rolls, kebabs, spring rolls, deep-fried samosas stuffed with potatoes, chicken and beef, deep-fried pakoras, nuggets of all types, and many other forms of breaded meat being sold in supermarkets.

● All bakery items, all kinds of breads made from refined flour, all kinds of pita breads, middle-eastern breads, naan, roti and so on.

● Ready-to-eat meals in packages and from fast-food restaurants.

● Soy milk, almond milk, all kinds of fruit juices and soft drinks.

● All kinds of soups and soup mixes being sold in supermarkets.

● Breakfast cereals of all kinds, being sold in supermarkets.

● All products made from whole milk such as cheese, whey, tofu from soy.

● Canned and frozen vegetables and fruits.

● All kinds of chips and snacks being sold in supermarkets and convenience stores.

● Processed peanuts, almonds, cashews with added salt being sold in plastic bags as snacks.

   Note: Dry-roasted raw peanuts, raw almonds, raw walnuts, raw cashews are whole foods.

● All kinds of sauces & dressings being served in restaurants or sold in supermarkets.

● Countless other items being sold in the stores everywhere.

REFINED FOODS [8, 9, 10]

Refined foods are not whole foods but processed foods that do not contain the original nutrients given by nature. Refined foods have been transformed and/or ground to their refined form from whole foods, and transported to supermarkets for distribution and direct consumption by customers. A refined food doesn't entirely contain its original nutrients in the whole food form, but is mixed with preservatives and/or artificial colors and flavors. **The altered texture and flavor make the body crave more of it. That is why your body wants more and more processed foods and refined foods.**

The human body does not process refined foods in the same way as whole foods, partially due to the decreased fiber content in refined foods. Refined foods are also generally many times higher in calories than whole foods. So your daily calorie consumption is a lot higher if you eat refined foods.

Examples of Refined Foods

A typical example is the STARCHY WHITE FLOUR OR ALL-PURPOSE WHITE FLOUR made from grains (mostly wheat, rice or both) by crushing them in a grinding machine. Refined foods lose fiber content after they are processed. Pizza dough, muffins, chips, Doritos, all bakery items such as pastries, cookies, donuts, cakes, ice cream cones, all kinds of breads, pita breads that are made from refined flour.

REASONS WHY YOU HAVE FAT IN THE BELLY

● You are tempted to overconsume flour-based foods because they look attractive to the eyes, are easier to chew in your mouth and are very tasty while chewing.

● When whole-kernel grains are crushed with machinery and refined to produce starch, 80 percent of the fiber is lost, and therefore the gut health suffers. [10]

● When you overconsume processed and refined foods, many heath hazards develop: food cravings, spiked blood sugar levels, metabolic slowdown, food allergies, acid-alkaline imbalances, inflammation, gastrointestinal-disorders or GI disorders such as acid reflux, heartburn, dyspepsia/indigestion, nausea and vomiting, peptic ulcer disease, abdominal pain syndrome, belching, bloating, flatulence, biliary tract disorders, gallbladder disorders and gallstone pancreatitis, and others. [10]

● Refined flours or foods made using refined flours act like sugars in the body, triggering weight gain and high blood sugar. People like to consume fancy food items made from refined flour because they taste better than whole foods and are easier to consume. Foods made from refined flour digest faster than whole foods, causing blood sugar spikes, which in turn demands an immediate spike in insulin levels in order to maintain normal blood sugar levels in the body. But when the pancreas fail to secrete enough insulin into the blood stream to transport the glucose, glucose gets accumulated in the blood stream resulting in type 2 diabetes. When people eat foods made from refined flour, they feel hungry again within 2 hours and eat more with developed cravings, causing the liver to manufacture fat in the belly. Obese and overweight people eventually develop type 2 diabetes. That is why if you eat whole foods, you would save your life and protect yourself from gaining weight and developing diabetes, sleep apnea, sleep disorders and other diseases.

NUTRIENTS ARE NEEDED FOR THE HUMAN BODY SURVIVAL [11]

In order to function properly, the human body must possess sufficient nutrients. A nutrient is a chemical or substance that an organism needs to survive and grow, or a nutrient is a substance taken from the environment and used in an organism's metabolism. The nutrients that are essential for the survival of human beings are: proteins, carbohydrates, fiber, fats, oils, vitamins, minerals and water. Nutrients are directly used to build and repair tissues, regulate the body's processes throughout the day. Nutrients are further converted into and used as energy for the living human body. The living human body needs nutrients for energy, to grow, and to repair itself. In addition, the human body needs water and fiber as well. You must consume the following seven types of nutrients every single day to be able to survive:

1. Water: About 70% of the human body is water. Water is required for the digestion, transport of nutrients in and out of your body's cells, lubrication, temperature regulation, etc.
2. Carbohydrates: Carbohydrates are the main source of energy.
3. Fats: Fats are a source of energy, and are used to repair cell parts.
4. Protein: Proteins are the building blocks making up body tissues, muscles, skin, and organs.
5. Vitamins: Vitamins enable chemical reactions in the body.
6. Minerals: Minerals aid enzyme function, and are utilized for the bone structure.
7. Fiber: Fiber is not digested by your body. Instead, it passes relatively intact through your stomach, small intestine and colon and moves out of your body. Fiber helps maintain bowel health, normalizes your bowel movement, helps control blood sugar levels, lowers cholesterol levels and aids achieving healthy weight and prevents colorectal cancer. Whole foods contain a lot of fiber whereas the refined and processed foods have already lost a lot of fiber content while being processed in manufacturing factories.

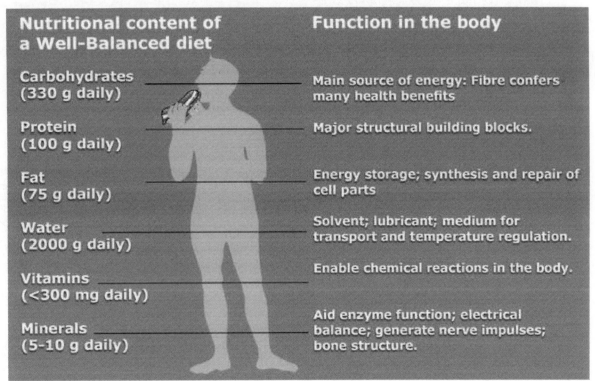

Nutritional content of a Well-Balanced diet	Function in the body
Carbohydrates (330 g daily)	Main source of energy: Fibre confers many health benefits
Protein (100 g daily)	Major structural building blocks.
Fat (75 g daily)	Energy storage; synthesis and repair of cell parts
Water (2000 g daily)	Solvent; lubricant; medium for transport and temperature regulation.
Vitamins (<300 mg daily)	Enable chemical reactions in the body.
Minerals (5-10 g daily)	Aid enzyme function; electrical balance; generate nerve impulses; bone structure.

Figure 3.1 Different nutrients and their functions in the body.

SIMPLE CARBOHYDRATES Vs COMPLEX CARBOHYDRATES [12, 13]

Carbohydrates are a major source of energy that your body requires. Almost all foods "except meats, chicken, fish, egg whites, spices, oils, and water" are loaded with carbohydrates. Carbohydrates are made up of sugar, starch and fiber.

There are two types of carbohydrates: a. Simple Carbohydrates
b. Complex Carbohydrates

Table 3.1 Simple carbohydrates versus complex carbohydrates.

SIMPLE CARBOHYDRATES	COMPLEX CARBOHYDRATES
Simple carbohydrates are sugary food items with little or no fiber that digest quickly and raise blood sugar levels. All processed foods and foods made from refined flour are simple carbohydrates, and demand a lot of insulin to transport glucose into the blood stream. If the pancreas fail to secrete insulin according to the demand, the glucose buildup in the blood stream could result in type 2 diabetes. High glucose levels are also a cause for fat in the belly. Examples: raw sugar, brown sugar, all bakery items made by adding tons of sugar, refined flour and butter such as cookies, biscuits, muffins, cakes, candies, white bread, pie, pizza dough, breakfast sugary cereals, sodas, fruit juices, etc. 🖐 you should deliberately identify and avoid simple carbohydrates in your diet, and consume only complex carbohydrates.	Complex carbohydrates are non-sugary food items with a lot of fiber along with vitamins & minerals that digest slower without any glucose spikes. All raw foods that are unprocessed and unrefined, contain complex carbohydrates. There are two types of complex carbohydrates: (i) Fibrous Foods (ii) Starchy Foods Fiber is essential for bowel movement, and lowers cholesterol levels. **Examples of Fibrous Foods:** whole grains, vegetables, raw fruits, beans, nuts & seeds. **Examples of Starchy Foods:** potatoes, legumes, whole wheat bread, raw cereal, oats, kidney beans, chick peas, rice, wheat, quinoa, etc. 🖐 You should wisely include complex carbohydrates in your diet. All Whole Foods contain complex carbohydrates.

Table 3.2 Good carbohydrates versus bad carbohydrates.

GOOD CARBOHYDRATES	BAD CARBOHYDRATES
• Complex carbs.	• Simple carbs.
• Digest slowly.	• Digest fast and raise blood sugar level.
• Prolonged energy.	• Short energy spike.
• High in fiber.	• Low in fiber.
• You feel full longer.	• You become hungry again.
• Natural sugar and low calories.	• Added sugar and more calories.
• Demand low levels of insulin.	• Demand higher insulin levels with spike in blood sugar.
• Used directly for the energy.	• Some are converted into fat cells.
• Low glycemic index.	• High glycemic index.
• Help with weight loss.	• Cause uncontrollable weight gain.

LIST OF VEGETABLES & GREENS (WHOLE FOODS) FOR EVERY DAY EATING

Consume a variety of healthy vegetables and greens so that your body would get enough vitamins, minerals and fiber. Change the combination of vegetables and greens every day. You should prepare your egg-white omelet every day with different vegetables and greens. Some of these greens such as Kale, Spinach, Mustard Green, Chard should be added directly into the vegetables while making egg-white omelet. And some of the other greens such as Microgreens, Romaine, Iceberg, Alfalfa Sprouts and Beets can be eaten outside the plate to add nutritional value to your meal. It is important that you should watch the calories being consumed, and limit the quantity of vegetables and greens being consumed in every meal so that you meet the requirements of the weight-loss plan. In other words, do not overconsume these food items. Purchase and eat only "organic vegetables and greens" and wash them thoroughly before cooking and eating. And more importantly do not store these vegetables and greens for more than a week at home. If you do store them for more than a week, they could lose nutritional value. Make sure that you have eaten by covering most of these vegetables and greens, listed below, at least once every single week.

Table 3.3 List of vegetables & greens (whole foods) for every day eating.

LIST OF VEGETABLES AND GREENS (PREFERABLY ORGANIC)	
1. Kale, Chard, Collard Greens	31. Tomatoes (all kinds)
2. Fennel, Leeks, Broccoli Rabe (Rapini)	32. Lemons & Limes
3. Spinach, Curry Leaves	
	33. Parsley, Cilantro
4. Broccoli, Romanesco	34. Microgreens
5. Cauliflower	(nutrient levels are 6 times higher)
6. Mushrooms (all kinds)	35. Basil Herb
7. Egg Plant (all kinds)	36. Arugula
8. Onions (Yellow, Red & White)	37. Dandelion Green
9. Green Onions	38. Mustard Green, Mint Leaves
10. Scallions	39. Alfalfa Sprouts & Other Sprouts
11. Bell Peppers (Green, Red & Yellow)	40. Head Lettuce
12. Cucumber and Zucchini	41. Green Leaf Lettuce
13. Long English Cukes	42. Red Leaf Lettuce
14. Bok Choy & Goi Lan (Chinese)	43. Romaine Lettuce
	44. Butter Lettuce
15. Brussels Sprouts	45. Boston Butterhead
16. Asparagus	46. Iceberg Lettuce
17. Okra	47. Watercress, Dill
18. Green Long Beans/Yardlong Beans	
19. Peas	48. Sweet Corn (limited quantity)
20. Radishes	49. Russet Potatoes (limited quantity)
21. Cabbage (Green & Red)	50. White Potatoes (limited quantity)
22. Carrots	51. Red Potatoes (limited quantity)
23. Celery	52. Little Potatoes (limited quantity)
24. Butternut Squash	53. Sweet Potatoes (limited quantity)
25. Acorn Squash, Squash Carnival	54. Yams (limited quantity)
26. Kabocha	
27. Pumpkins	55. Beets (fresh, soft & juicy)
	56. Purple Top Turnips (limited quantity)
28. Garlic	57. Rutabagas, Daikon (limited quantity)
29. Ginger	58. Parsnips (limited quantity)
30. Horse Raddish	59. Artichokes (limited quantity)
	60. Celery roots (limited quantity)

REFERENCES

1. Processed Foods Vs Whole Foods.
   http://www.naturalnews.com/022175_food_foods_health.html

2. List of Raw Foods.
   https://news.therawfoodworld.com/whole-foods-list/

3. Whole Vs Processed Foods.
   https://www.azumio.com/blog/nutrition/whole-food-vs-processed

4. A list of Processed Foods.
   http://www.healthy-eating-politics.com/processed-foods.html

5. There is proof: Processed Foods are harder to digest and make the people fat and cause diseases.
   http://foodbabe.com/2012/08/01/theres-proof-processed-foods-are-harder-to-digest/

6. Processed Meats are too dangerous for human consumption.
   https://www.institutefornaturalhealing.com/2015/07/processed-meats-declared-too-dangerous-for-human-consumption/

7. World Cancer Research Fund International.
   http://wcrf.org/int/research-we-fund/continuous-update-project-cup
   Work is underway to develop a methodology for systematically reviewing human and animal mechanistic studies on the link between diet, nutrition, physical activity and the development and progression of different cancers.

8. The difference between Processed Foods and Refined Foods.
   http://www.trishamandes.com/blog/2014/12/8/the-difference-between-processed-and-refined-foods

9. Whole Foods Vs Processed Foods Vs Refined Foods.
   http://www.heathernicholds.com/nutrition/whole-processed-refined-foods

10. The truth about grains: Whole and Refined.
    https://experiencelife.com/article/the-truth-about-refined-grains/

11. Nutrients are needed for the survival of the human body (Google search).
    https://www.google.ca/search?q=human+body+need+nutrients+carbohydrates+fats+protein&biw=1280&bih=890&tbm=isch&tbo=u&source=univ&sa=X&ved=0ahUKEwixpaaZ8PzQAhVriVQKHZYPC3QQsAQIJg#imgrc=1c-RrhToluHHaM%3A

12. Simple Carbohydrates Vs Complex Carbohydrates.
    http://www.healthline.com/health/food-nutrition/simple-carbohydrates-complex-carbohydrates#1

13. A Guide to Complex Carbohydrates.
    http://www.livestrong.com/article/27398-list-complex-carbohydrates-foods/

14. Dr. Andrew Weil's Video on Nutritional Value of Organic Foods.
    https://www.llacuna.org/dr-weil-on-organic-food/?gclid=Cj0KEQiAy53DBRCo4en29Zvcla0BEiQAVIDcc1Le5F8_UF5Ez9uYujYzFol9JiKD1F5lSzau2vdt4PYaAs_j8P8HAQ

15. Nutritional Value of Organic Food.
    http://www.eostreorganics.co.uk/

CHAPTER 4   APPLE CIDER VINEGAR

TABLE OF CONTENTS

APPLE CIDER VINEGAR

Some people believe that Apple Cider Vinegar, if consumed continuously every day just before meals, helps in weight loss to some extent. Many people believe that Apple Cider Vinegar is a hunger suppressant and digestion promoter. If consumed before eating 2 to 3 times a day, it acts as a hunger suppressant and makes you feel full, and improves the digestion process.

History of Vinegar as a Health Food [1, 2, 3]
In French, vinegar means sour wine (vinaigre = vinegar, vin=wine, aigre = sour).
5000 BC: The Babylonians produced both wine and vinegar from the fruit of the date palm and used vinegar as a health food and as a pickling agent.
3000 BC: Vinegar residues have been found in ancient Egyptian urns.
1200 BC: The Chinese record books showed the production and use of vinegar.
400 BC: Evidence suggested that, in ancient Greece, Hippocrates prescribed apple cider vinegar mixed with honey for a variety of ailments.

Vinegar Vs Apple Cider Vinegar [4, 5, 6]

Table 4.1 Vinegar versus apple cider vinegar.

Vinegar	Apple Cider Vinegar (ACV)
● Vinegar is a clear, refined, distilled, filtered and pasteurized liquid without any mother culture settled at the bottom of the liquid. ● Vinegar contains about 5 to 20% acetic acid and the remaining percentage being the water and traces of a variety of chemicals. Vinegar is used extensively as a cleaning agent. Vinegar is used a lot in cooking, pickling, salad dressing at home and in restaurants. Vinegar is also used as a disinfectant that destroys bacteria.	● Apple Cider Vinegar, also called ACV, has a brownish-gold color, unrefined, unpasteurized and unfiltered liquid with the mother. The mother, a cloudy layer settles at the bottom, and is rich in vitamins, enzymes and amino acids. So always shake the bottle before pouring into a tablespoon. ● Apple Cider Vinegar is made from cider or apple must, and contains about 5 to 6% of acetic acid along with other acids, chemicals and water. ♦ Apple Cider vinegar has been used as a daily tonic for myriad heath issues such as: weight gain (acts as an appetite suppressant due to pectin), urinary track infection (UTI), high blood pressure, diabetes (lowers glucose levels and keeps insulin levels low), high cholesterol, allergies, aging, cancer, digestion, common cold; ACV cleanses the body off toxins through the skin, assists in the breakdown of protein and iron from food in the stomach, being a thermogenic agent, it increases the body temperature, helps reduce acne, blemishes, and oily skin and has other benefits. ♦ Apple Cider Vinegar is what many people use to clean linoleum floors. ♦ Apple Cider Vinegar has been used to get rid of dandruff. ♦ Apple cider Vinegar has the ability to get rid of dog and cat urine odor. ♦ Apple Cider Vinegar has been used to treat sunburns and insect bites.

HOW VINEGAR IS MADE BY YEAST & BACTERIAL FERMENTATION

Vinegar is made by fermentation commercially or at home. By combining fruit pieces, water, sugar and a fermenting agent (starter culture) such as yeast or whey. Yeasts are eukaryotic, single-celled microorganisms classified as members of the fungus kingdom. Vinegar is produced in a slow process by storing the liquid mixture in glass jars with the openings sealed by means of a porous cloth or a filter paper so that the jar is always exposed to air and is in contact with oxygen, and by allowing the liquid to stay in a dark place from several weeks to several months.

The chemical reactions take place in a two-step process in which the glucose of the sugar solution reacts with the fermenting agent yeast to form ethyl alcohol (ethanol) along with a byproduct called carbon dioxide [8]. The ethyl alcohol (ethanol) in turn reacts with the oxygen from air to form acetic acid and water, which is the final product called vinegar [7].

Step 1
Glucose + Yeast Enzyme = Ethanol or Ethyl Alcohol + Carbon Dioxide (CO_2)

$$(C_6H_{12}O_6) + \text{Yeast Enzyme} \rightarrow 2\,(CH_3CH_2OH) + 2\,CO_2$$

Step 2
Ethanol / Ethyl Alcohol + Oxygen = Acetic Acid + Water

$$CH_3CH_2OH + O_2 \rightarrow CH_3COOH + H_2O$$

5% to 20% of vinegar is acetic acid and the rest of it is water and traces of other chemicals. To accelerate the production of vinegar, the bacterial culture (usually the mother of vinegar) is added in the second step. Apple cider vinegar is made from apple cider or apple must, instead of apples pieces, and has a brownish-gold color.

Vinegar has been produced and consumed throughout human history, from fruits such as apples, grapes, sugar cane, coconut, raspberries, kiwifruit, kombucha, malt, palm, pomegranate, sherries, raisin, rice, wheat, millet and many others. [7, 9]

How Organic Apple Cider Vinegar With Mother is Made at Home [10, 11, 12, 13]
Fill three-fourth of a glass jar with roughly chopped and cleaned organic ripe apple pieces. Do not use a metal jar as the acid would react with the metal). Crush the apples pieces until they become apple pulp. Prepare a sugar solution by dissolving 1 tablespoon of organic cane sugar per 1 cup of purified or distilled water. Prepare as much sugar solution as needed to fill three-fourth of the glass jar. Pour the sugar solution into the glass jar 3/4 full, and mix the apple pulp with a long spoon or stirrer. Cover the glass jar by means of a cheesecloth or coffee-filter paper so that the apples would be able to breath. Secure the top of the glass jar firmly with a thread or rubber band. Then place the glass jar in a dark place, most commonly underneath the kitchen cabinet.

The glass jar should not be exposed to sunlight or high room temperatures. The room temperature should be between 60 °F and 80 °F (15.5 °C and 26.6 °C) to attain successful yeast fermentation. Yeast fermentation is completed in 3 to 4 weeks.

After 3 to 4 weeks, open the glass jar and strain its contents. Remove the apple pieces and return the liquid back to the glass jar. Cover it with a new cheesecloth or a new coffee-filter paper. Secure the top again with a thread or a rubber band, and leave it in a dark place for another 3 to 4 more weeks, but remember to stir it once every few days. Also taste a few drops to see if it is sour enough. Once the liquid has reached the desired tartness (it tastes sour), you could call it the "Apple Cider Vinegar' and start consuming it. At this time you would find a cloudy layer settled at the bottom of the jar. It is called mother which is rich in enzymes. If you do not pasteurize it and do not filter out the mother settled at the bottom, you can call it "organic apple cider vinegar with the mother, unpasteurized and unfiltered," which is the best final product to consume.

Two Brand Names for Organic Apple Cider Vinegar

Organic Apple Cider Vinegar is being manufactured and distributed worldwide under two major companies BRAGG & Omega. BRAGG'S Apple Cider Vinegar is currently the most popular one, and is available in all health food stores and in some grocery stores as well.

BRAGG ORGANIC RAW UNFILTERED APPLE CIDER VINEGAR With The Mother Unpasteurized and Naturally Gluten-Free	OMEGA NUTRITION ORGANIC APPLE CIDER VINEGAR With Mother, Unfiltered & Unpasteurized with 5% Acitic Acid
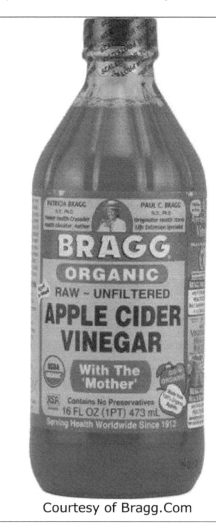 Courtesy of Bragg.Com	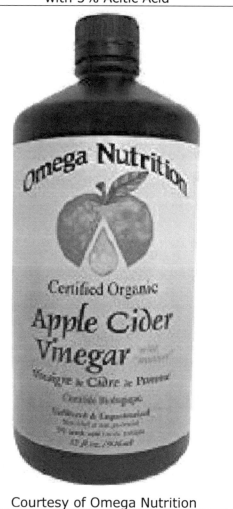 Courtesy of Omega Nutrition

Figure 4.1 Organic apple cider vinegar available to purchase.

67

**HOW TO CONSUME ORGANIC APPLE CIDER VINEGAR
With Mother, Unpasteurized & Unfiltered**

- Always drink Apple Cider Vinegar (AVC) in a glass cup with a straw.
  If you drink ACV without a straw, the acid content would damage your teeth.
- Do not use a metal container when you drink Apple Cider Vinegar.
  The acid content of ACV could react with the metal container.
- Mix 2 to 3 tablespoons of Apple Cider Vinegar (ACV) in a glass cup of
  warm purified water, and sip it before meals, 2 to 3 times a day.
- Always rinse your mouth immediately after consuming ACV,
  else the traces of acid in your mouth could damage your teeth.

- You can add a pinch of Cayenne Pepper (if you like the flavor),
  as it neutralizes the acidity, and adds flavor to your drink.
  pH of Apple Cider Vinegar ≈ 3.0; pH of Cayenne Pepper ≈ 8.5
- You can also add lemon juice or lime juice to improve the taste.
- You can also add honey to further improve the taste, though honey is not
  recommended when you are trying to lose weight.

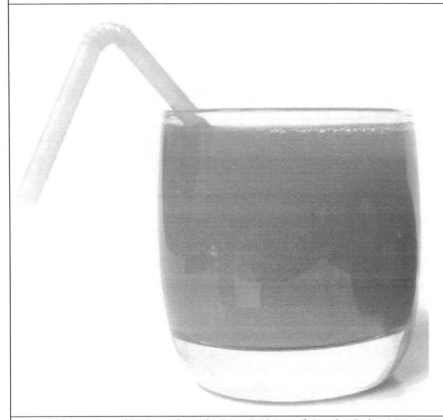

A Glass Cup (250 mL) with 2 to 3 tbsp of Apple Cider Vinegar + Purified Water +
A Pinch of Organic Cayenne Pepper. Always Sip It With a Straw.

Figure 4.2 How to consume organic apple cider vinegar.

LISTEN TO THE RESEARCHERS, HEALTH EXPERTS AND HEALTH WRITERS

1. How Does Apple Cider Vinegar Help You Lose Weight? [14]

Apple cider vinegar with the mother is loaded with vitamins, minerals, enzymes and amino acids. Its various enzymes aid in the digestion process. Apples, oranges and grapefruit contain both soluble and insoluble fiber along with a particular form of fiber called pectin. The pectin fiber is believed to suppress hunger and makes a person feel full upon consumption. One medium apple with the skin contains approximately 4 g of fiber and 1.5 g of pectin. The pH of apple cider vinegar is listed as 2.9, which means it is very acidic. The acid content of apple cider vinegar along with pectin fiber is believed to stimulate the digestion process, which is essential for the synthesis of growth hormones. The fiber content of pectin is also responsible for lowering cholesterol levels. Growth hormones are responsible for the breakdown of fats during the digestion process, and the same hormones keep the metabolism going while we rest after our meals. This is why we must consume two tablespoons of apple cider vinegar diluted in a cup of water, using a straw, just before our evening meal every day. The combined effect of pectin and the acidity of apple cider vinegar would help lose weight.

Acetic acid found in the apple cider vinegar helps release iron in the food you eat and makes it more available to be a building block for the oxygen-carrying hemoglobin and oxygen-attracting myoglobin. Oxygen is an essential component for burning energy in the body. As apple cider vinegar increases iron utilization and energy consumption in the body, you should encourage yourself to consume apple cider vinegar on a daily basis if you want to lose weight.

Apple cider vinegar is also a great source of potassium (potassium supplements are recommended in weight loss programs), which helps balance the salt content in the food consumed. Salt being a flavor enhancer, if consumed excessively, not only increases the water weight you carry in your fatty belly but also tempts you to eat more salty foods, and further adds pounds to your fat. So if you could cut the salt intake in your diet and substitute it with apple cider vinegar instead, experts believe it would help you lose weight reasonably.

2. How Pectin in Vegetables & Fruits Helps in Weight Loss [15, 16, 17]

One medium-size apple with the skin contains approximately 4.0 g of fiber and 1.5 g of pectin. Pectin being a soluble fiber absorbs water and forms a viscous mass that expands in the stomach, making you feel full. The stretch receptor in the stomach and small intestine triggers signals to the brain, informing that the stomach is full. The brain then orders to release the pertinent hormones and the body feels a sense of satiety. The viscous mass created by pectin also delays the movement of finely crushed meal by passing very slowly through the stomach, small intestine and large intestine. This kind of slow movement of viscous mass extends the feeling of fullness in the stomach, thereby making you eat less, which contributes to weight loss. Moreover pectin adds moisture to the stool and, by mixing with the available bacteria in the large intestine, generates energy to be used by the large intestine.

It is believed that pectin combats leptin resistance thereby promoting weight loss. Apples, oranges and grapefruit contain pectin fiber, which suppress appetite by tricking the brain into believing that your stomach is full.

Carrots, cucumbers, tomatoes and many other vegetables help suppress hunger by offering low calories at the same time. Raw or semi-cooked vegetables and the aforementioned fruits (apples, oranges and grapefruit) contain the most important nutrients your body requires, and they also increase the metabolic rate.

Other fruits such as gooseberries, plums, quince, guavas, strawberries, grapes and cherries also contain pectin in small quantities. Pectin is beneficial for digestion and in controlling cholesterol. The high fiber content of vegetables and fruits contributes to weight loss. So incorporate them into your diet.

3. Apple Cider Vinegar Improves Blood Sugar Regulation and Speeds Up Weight Loss [18, 19, 20, 21, 22, 23] The daily intake of apple cider vinegar may promote the antiglycemic effect and suppression of carbohydrate synthesis, resulting in the regulation of satiety and/or appetite. The end result could be weight loss. [19]

In Japan 155 obese people participated in a research to see the effect of apple cider vinegar on weight loss. The research data revealed that there was a significant reduction of viscerial fat, body mass index (BMI) and serum triglyceride levels of those obese people. [20]

The research study also reported that weight loss may have been caused from the stimulation of fecal bile acid excretion. They also reported that as apple cider vinegar has the ability of detoxification, the overall health of the liver improved significantly. [21]

The Diabetes Journal published a study in 2007 reporting the effects of vinegar on waking hyperglycemia in type 2 diabetics. [22]

When some individuals consumed 2 tablespoons of apple cider vinegar, they noticed a 4-6% reduction in their fasting glucose levels. Another study reported that some women had 55% reduction in their blood glucose levels following a morning meal containing vinegar. [23]

4. Three Ways Apple Cider Vinegar Benefits Weight Loss, NaturalNews.com. (n.d.) [24, 25, 26, 27, 28, 29, 30, 31]
Recent research shows that there are at least three ways in which the traditional healers were on the right track when it comes to weight loss.

a. A 2006 review article in the "Medscape Journal of Medicine" concluded that vinegar may have a role in blood sugar control and appetite suppression. Other studies show vinegar may also promote weight loss by preventing fat accumulation through its impact on insulin secretion.

b. Animal studies offer further proof of the value of drinking vinegar to lose weight. Scientists in Pakistan mixed apple cider vinegar with food given to diabetic and non-diabetic rats. The result was significantly lower LDL and higher HDL cholesterol in the non-diabetic rats. Similarly, the diabetic rats enjoyed significantly lower triglyceride levels and raised levels of HDL cholesterol. In a 2009 study, which used mice as subjects, acetic acid (the main ingredient in vinegar) was associated with reduced liver lipids and less fat accumulation.

c. In a 2005 study in the "European Journal of Clinical Nutrition," scientists fed bread plus low, medium or high amounts of vinegar to twelve healthy subjects, while the control group ate plain bread. Those who received the vinegar felt fuller than the control group, and the effect increased with the amount of vinegar ingested. While vinegar soaked bread may not be your favorite dish, you might try sipping vinegar in water along with your meal or having a salad dressed with vinegar and oil. Be sure to brush your teeth after sipping vinegar as it can be hard on tooth enamel.

d. Individuals with type 2 diabetes or who are pre-diabetic may benefit from vinegar's apparent ability to stabilize glucose. A 2007 study reported in "Diabetes Care" followed 11 people diagnosed with type 2 diabetes, but who were not taking insulin. Every night for 3 nights they ingested either 2 tablespoons of apple cider vinegar or water plus some cheese. The results showed drinking vinegar at bedtime had a significant and favorable impact on waking, or fasting glucose concentrations even among the subjects who were taking hypoglycemic medications during the study.

e. By promoting stable blood sugar, vinegar may help prevent the sugar crashes that encourage you to wolf down the nearest source of carbohydrates, shooting your blood sugar back up and starting the cycle all over again. In the 2005 study of vinegar and satiety, the scientists also evaluated blood samples to determine vinegar's impact on glucose and insulin levels. The low and intermediate vinegar groups had significantly lowered blood glucose levels at 15 and 30 minutes, which continued to be measurable at 90 minutes for the high vinegar group. Similarly, the intermediate group enjoyed lower insulin levels at 15 minutes, the high group at 30 minutes.

f. In a 2004 study in "Diabetes Care", insulin-resistant individuals who drank vinegar and water followed by a meal enjoyed significantly improved insulin sensitivity compared to a control group. The study authors concluded that vinegar's effects may be similar to those of some popular diabetes drugs. Of course given the connection between insulin levels and fat storage, these results support vinegar's use as a fat-burning food.

5. What Does Apple Cider Vinegar (AVC) Do To Make You Lose Weight? [32]
ACV taps into several physiological mechanisms that support healthy weight loss:
a. ACV acts as an appetite suppressor.
b. ACV controls blood sugar levels.
c. ACV prevents fat accumulation.
d. ACV has an impact on insulin secretion.
e. ACV detoxifies the body.

6. Ten Uses of Apple Cider Vinegar for Great Health [33]
 Apple Cider Vinegar (AVC) has the following 10 health benefits:
a. AVC provides better nutrition absorption.
b. AVC improves digestion.
c. AVC eases muscle cramps.
d. AVC kills fungus.
e. An AVC rinse can make the hair healthy and shiny.
f. AVC can whiten your teeth (wash your teeth immediately or teeth can be damaged.)
g. AVC can clean kitchen surfaces, sinks, windows, mirrors and kitchen appliances.
h. AVC can be used to remove bad odor.
i. AVC can unclog and clean your shower head.
j. AVC can be used as flea repellent for your pets.

7. Six Proven Benefits of Apple Cider Vinegar [34]

Apple Cider Vinegar has the following 6 proven health benefits:

a. AVC is High in acetic acid, which has potent biological effects.
b. AVC can kill many types of bacteria.
c. AVC lowers blood sugar levels and fights diabetes.
d. AVC helps you lose weight by making you feel full.
e. AVC lowers cholesterol and reduces the risk for heart disease.
f. AVC may have protective effects against cancer.

8. Seven Side Effects of Apple Cider Vinegar [35]

Do Not Overconsume Apple Cider Vinegar!

Apple Cider Vinegar (AVC) has to be consumed in the right dosage and with appropriate caution. You should make sure that it suits your body or it may have negative effects on your body. If you overconsume apple cider vinegar without researching its effects on yourself, the following 7 side effects are possible:

a. AVC may cause delayed stomach emptying.
b. AVC may have digestive side effect such as indigestion.
c. AVC may cause low potassium levels, resulting in bone loss.
d. AVC may cause erosion of tooth enamel.
e. AVC may cause throat burns.
f. AVC may cause skin burns.
g. AVC may cause prescription-drug interactions.

9. Can You Lose Weight Taking Apple Cider Vinegar Pills? [36]

According to a report published in the Journal of American Dietetic Association in 2005, apple cider vinegar in pill form may not contain what it says on the bottle. So do not trust the tablets, pills or capsules being sold in shops. Instead, it is better recommended that you consume organic apple cider vinegar with the mother (the liquid in a bottle), unpasteurized and unfiltered to get maximum benefits.

THIS IS WHAT I HAVE DONE

▶ I firmly believe that apple cider vinegar contributed to my weight loss program in some way or the other.

🌑 I dissolve 2 to 3 tablespoons of apple cider vinegar (I shake the bottle before using it) along with a pinch of cayenne pepper in a cup of warm water, and sip it by means of a STRAW (I know that I should never drink apple cider vinegar with water directly without a straw or it would harm my teeth). I do so 2 to 3 times a day, just before my pre-workout meal and my post-workout meal. Sometimes I take it a third time just before my evening meal. That means I consume more than 6 tablespoons a day. I sip and finish the whole cup very quickly within a minute, just before eating my meal. I did not have any serious side effects as I have been consuming it every day for the last 3 to 4 months. When I started it in the beginning, I faced frequent urination problem. But I did not care as I drink a lot of water during the day and my body had been burning fat. So I needed to urinate a lot in order to flush out the waste being generated by fat metabolism.

🌑 After I started taking apple cider vinegar in September 2016, within a month, my digestion and therefore my metabolism improved. My stubborn belly fat began melting away and I started losing pounds of my excess weight and inches of belly fat around my waist. My blood sugar levels stabilized (I have been a serious insulin-dependent diabetic for over 35 years), my hemoglobin A1c dropped to an all-time LOW 5.0%, my LDL cholesterol dropped close to the lower end of normal (all-time LOW), my triglycerides test was found to be the all-time lowest. I had extremely impressive blood test results on the diabetes panel on October 1st, 2016. Since then, I have continued taking apple cider vinegar two to three times every day. My total consumption is more than 6 tablespoons a day.

🌑 All the following factors contributed to my weight loss:
The low-calorie and low-fat or zero-fat self-prevention diet that I created with whole foods (mostly vegetables), egg whites, apple cider vinegar, Kamut Puffs that I have been eating as an in-between meals snack, daily exercise for 60 to 90 minutes and 16 cups (4 liters) of purified water per day. In addition, this weight-loss program requires very high willpower, very high self-discipline and the strong desire to succeed in order to avoid eating out, consuming junk foods (containing processed foods and refined foods) in restaurants and to avoid cheating my own diet plan. All of the aforementioned factors individually and collectively contributed to my weight loss and eventually my sleep apnea has been reversed after losing 40 pounds of body weight and 12 inches around the waist.

THIS IS WHAT YOU SHOULD DO

🌑 Apple cider vinegar may not directly help you lose weight. So do not get frustrated and give up on it. Even if it does not yield positive results immediately, apple cider vinegar would suppress your hunger and in turn make you feel fuller and thus you will eat less. It will help in the digestion process and improve your overall health with the vitamins, minerals, enzymes and amino acids present in the mother of the apple cider vinegar. Always shake the bottle before you use it so that you consume at least a little of the mother of the apple cider vinegar every time.

🌑 You may face very common side effect such as "frequent urination" when you first try apple cider vinegar. But don't worry! Be persistent! After a couple of days or after a week, the frequent urination will stop. If you are affected by any side effect of apple cider vinegar, lower the dosage but do not discontinue. Instead of 3 times a day, take apple cider vinegar twice a day or once a day. Instead of mixing 2 tablespoons of apple cider vinegar in a cup of water each time, mix only 1 tablespoon of apple cider vinegar, but continue like that until you get used to it, and until you improve your overall health.

● Each time add a pinch of cayenne pepper, if you could, along with the apple cider vinegar in the cup of warm water, it would neutralize the acidity. You would feel better when you sip it and during the digestion process. Eventually with some trying, you would get used to it. If cayenne pepper does not suit you, skip it or try honey instead.

● Use trial and error to find out for yourself the right dosage of apple cider vinegar for you. You should check if you are able to consume it 3 times a day, 2 times a day or just 1 time a day. Even one tablespoon a day could significantly improve your health. One tablespoon a day would not cause you any side effects. Gradually figure which time of the day, morning, afternoon or evening suits you best to consume that 1 tablespoon of apple cider vinegar. Try all possibilities to learn your optimal dosage or tolerance to apple cider vinegar (how many tablespoons you could consume at a given time during a given day without feeling its side effects).

● REMEMBER: You should always use a straw when you take apple cider vinegar with water, else the acid content of it would damage your teeth.

● Don't give up apple cider vinegar immediately. Instead lower the dosage if it tastes bad or if it causes digestive problems, throat burns, or other problems.

● Once you are accustomed to apple cider vinegar, you would love it, and would be able to take advantage of its multiple health benefits discussed in this chapter. It would work wonders for your health in a long run, if not in a short time.

● Do not take apple cider vinegar tablets, pills or capsules as the health experts cautioned that they were found to be unreliable and untrustworthy. [36]

REFERENCES

1. Vinegar History.
http://www.apple-cider-vinegar-benefits.com/vinegar-history.html

2. Vinegar Tips: History.
http://vinegartips.com/history/

3. What does apple cider vinegar not do? What can it do for your body?
http://www.pacificcollege.edu/news/blog/2015/04/25/what-does-apple-cider-vinegar-not-do?mailaddress=true&mailaddress=true&mailaddress=true

4. The Benefits of Apple Cider Vinegar.
http://www.getridofthings.com/glossary/the-benefits-of-apple-cider-vinegar/

5. Apple Cider Vinegar Health Benefits/Results.
https://www.reddit.com/r/Fitness/comments/14buzp/apple_cider_vinegar_health_benefitsresults/

6. Exposing the Scam: Health Benefits of Apple Cider Vinegar by Dr. T. Colin Campell With pH Values and Calories of All Types of Vinegars
https://www.superfoodly.com/health-benefits-of-apple-cider-vinegar-uses/

7. Vinegar (from Wikipedia).
https://en.wikipedia.org/wiki/Vinegar

8. What is the Chemical Reaction between Yeast and Sugar?
https://www.reference.com/science/chemical-reaction-between-yeast-sugar-fb04a3807cdd557f#

9. How to Ferment Fruit to Make Alcohol.
https://www.leaf.tv/articles/how-to-ferment-fruit-to-make-alcohol/

10. How to make apple cider vinegar at home.
http://wellnessmama.com/124169/make-apple-cider-vinegar/

11. How to make your own apple cider vinegar.
http://www.naturallivingideas.com/homemade-apple-cider-vinegar/

12. Apple Cider Vinegar Recipe - Make your own vinegar.
http://www.pickyourown.org/AppleCiderVinegarRecipe.php

13. How to make apple cider vinegar.
https://www.earthclinic.com/remedies/how_to_make_apple_cider_vinegar.html

14. How Does Apple Cider Vinegar Help You Lose Weight.
     Posted by Cynthia Holzapfel | 743 Comments.
http://www.vegkitchen.com/tips/healthy-eating-tips-tips/how-does-apple-cider-vinegar-work-to-help-you-lose-weight/

15. Pectin & Weight Loss, Posted by SANDI BUSCH Last Updated: Oct 12, 2015.
http://www.livestrong.com/article/314710-pectin-weight-loss/

16. Pectin Helps Leptin Resistance (by HealwithFood.Org).
http://www.healwithfood.org/articles/pectin-leptin-resistance.php

17. Fruits That Reduce Your Appetite
http://www.diethealthclub.com/diet-and-weight-loss/fruits-to-reduce-appetite.html

18. Apple Cider Vinegar improves blood sugar regulation and speeds up weight loss,
    Posted by Dr. David Jockers, March 18, 2015.
http://www.naturalnews.com/049034_apple_cider_vinegar_blood_sugar_weight_loss.html

19. Effect and mechanisms of action of vinegar on glucose metabolism, lipid profile, and
body weight. Petsiou EI, Mitrou PI, et al, Oxford University Press Journals. 2014 Oct; 651-
661. DOI: 10.1111/nure.12125.
https://www.ncbi.nlm.nih.gov/pubmed/25168916

20. Vinegar intake reduces body weight, body fat mass, and serum triglyceride levels in
obese Japanese subjects, Kondo T, et al., Biosci Biotechnol Biochem. 2009 Apr; 73(8):
1837-1843. DOI: 10.127//bbb.90231.
https://www.ncbi.nlm.nih.gov/pubmed/19661687

21. Dietary acetic acid reduces serum cholesterol and triacylglycerols in rats fed a
cholesterol-rich diet.Takashi Fushimi, Kazuhito Suruga, Yoshifumi Oshima, Momoko
Fukiharu, Yoshinori Tsukamoto and Toshinao Goda, British Journal of Nutrition. 2006 May;
95:916-924. DOI: 10.1079/BJN20061740.
https://www.cambridge.org/core/services/aop-cambridge-
core/content/view/S000711450600119X

22. Vinegar ingestion at bedtime moderates waking glucose concentrations in adults with
well-controlled type 2 diabetes.
White AM, Johnston CS, Diabetes Care. 2007 Nov; 30:2814-2815. PMID: 17712024
https://www.ncbi.nlm.nih.gov/pubmed/17712024

23. Vinegar and peanut products as complementary foods to reduce postprandial glycemia.
Johnston CS, Buller AJ, J Am Diet Assoc. 2005 Dec;105:1939-1942. PMID: 16321601
https://www.ncbi.nlm.nih.gov/pubmed/16321601

SCIENTIFIC RESEARCH PUBLICATIONS
24. Three ways apple cider vinegar benefits weight loss – NaturalNews.com. (n.d.).
Retrieved from
http://www.naturalnews.com/033745_apple_cider_vinegar_weight_loss.html

25. Vinegar: Medicinal Uses and Antiglycemic Effect, MedGenMed Journal, 2006.
https://www.ncbi.nlm.nih.gov/pmc/articles/PMC1785201/

26. Vinegar Consumption Increases Insulin-Stimulated Glucose Uptake by the Forearm
Muscle in Humans with Type 2 Diabetes, Journal of Diabetes Research, 2015.
https://www.ncbi.nlm.nih.gov/pmc/articles/PMC4438142/

27. Vinegar supplementation lowers glucose and insulin responses and increases satiety after a bread meal in healthy subjects.
https://www.ncbi.nlm.nih.gov/pubmed/16015276
http://www.nature.com/ejcn/journal/v59/n9/full/1602197a.html

28. Vinegar Ingestion at Bedtime Moderates Waking Glucose Concentrations in Adults With Well-Controlled Type 2 Diabetes.
http://care.diabetesjournals.org/content/30/11/2814.full

29. Vinegar Improves Insulin Sensitivity to a High-Carbohydrate Meal in Subjects With Insulin Resistance or Type 2 Diabetes.
http://care.diabetesjournals.org/content/27/1/281.full

30. Apple cider vinegar attenuates lipid profile in normal and diabetic rats.
https://www.ncbi.nlm.nih.gov/pubmed/19630216

31. Acetic acid upregulates the expression of genes for fatty acid oxidation enzymes in liver to suppress body fat accumulation.
https://www.ncbi.nlm.nih.gov/pubmed/19469536

32. HOW TO USE APPLE CIDER VENEGAR FOR WEIGHT LOSS?
What Does ACV Do To Make You Lose Weight?
http://www.healthyandnaturalworld.com/how-to-use-apple-cider-vinegar-for-weight-loss/
Posted by Jenny Hills, March 5, 2015.

33. Ten Uses for Apple Cider Vinegar for Great Health and At Home.
http://www.healthyandnaturalworld.com/10-uses-for-apple-cider-vinegar-for-great-health/
Posted by Amy Goodrich, Jan 10, 2014.

34. Six Proven Benefits of Apple Cider Vinegar, Posted by Kris Gunnars, BSc.
https://authoritynutrition.com/6-proven-health-benefits-of-apple-cider-vinegar/

35. Seven Side Effects of Too Much Apple Cider Vinegar, Posted by Franziska Spritzler, RD, CDE
https://authoritynutrition.com/apple-cider-vinegar-side-effects/

36. Can You Lose Weight Taking Apple Cider Vinegar Pills?, Posted by JILL CORLEONE, RDN, LD, Last Updated: Apr 27, 2016.
http://www.livestrong.com/article/290456-can-you-lose-weight-taking-apple-cider-vinegar-pills/

CHAPTER 5   PURIFIED WATER

TABLE OF CONTENTS

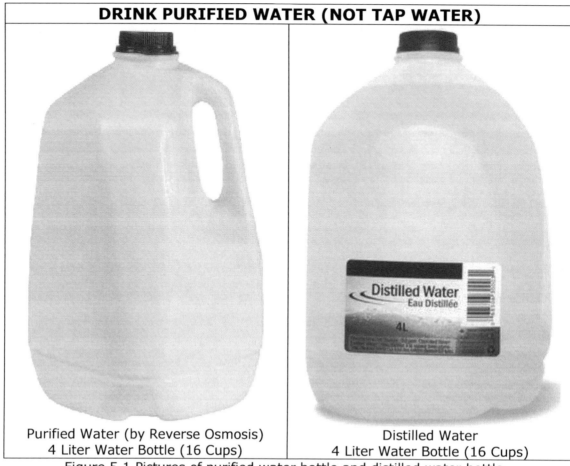

DRINK PURIFIED WATER (NOT TAP WATER)

Purified Water (by Reverse Osmosis) 4 Liter Water Bottle (16 Cups)	Distilled Water 4 Liter Water Bottle (16 Cups)

Figure 5.1 Pictures of purified water bottle and distilled water bottle.

THE IMPORTANCE OF WATER [1, 2, 18]

The human body needs water for its survival. About 70 to 75%% of the human body is made up of water. Two thirds of the earth's surface is covered by water, and it was abundantly clear that water is one of the prime elements responsible for life on earth. The only element more important than water for human body survival is oxygen. Listed below are the most important benefits of water:

◉ Water is beneficial and vital to the life of every human being, animal and plant. To feel fit and healthy, the human body should stay hydrated all the time. When you water your plants, you watch them glow taller and greener. Exactly like that, when you drink water, water acts on your body to grow and keeps you active and healthy.

◉ Every cell, tissue and organ in your body needs water to function correctly.

◉ Water is required in your stomach, small intestine and colon for the digestion, transportation and distribution of nutrients in and out of the body's cells, lubrication, temperature regulation, removal of wastes, etc. Water regulates body temperature precisely and aids digestion process. Large amount of water is needed to transport and digest solid foods. When you eat sold foods, you should drink a lot of water. Water is lost from your body when you urinate, sweat and even when you breath out. You should immediately replace lost water by drinking more and more water throughout the day.

Just listen to your body, and whenever your body demands, you must drink water.

● Water transports nutrients throughout the entire body, especially to the brain. About 85% of the brain is in the water that helps feed and cushion it.

● Every part of your body relies on ample hydration to function properly. Water lifts you up, opens your senses and makes you feel refreshed and ready to take on any activity, including even sleeping.

● Water lubricates and cushions your body's bones and joints. Water helps heal quickly the joint damages. Water helps maintain muscle tone as muscles are composed primarily of water. Even the fat contains about 20% of water.

● Water helps your kidneys and liver function properly and helps reduce the fat deposits. The kidneys need plenty of water to remove salt from the blood and to remove toxins and waste. Water lubricates all your organs so that they function at their best. Water also helps the blood from thickening.

How Much Water A Person Should Drink?
Health experts recommend that an adult must drink 8 glasses of water per day.
1 Glass = 1 Cup = 250 mL = 1/4 Liter.

But Extreme Weight Loss Contestants drink double that amount. That means they drink 16 cups or 4 Liters of water per day to achieve their weight loss goals.

I started drinking 16 cups or 4 Liters per day when I seriously began my weight loss program after I was diagnosed with sleep apnea in February 2015. Before that I was drinking only 8 cups of water per day. I now drink and finish the whole 4 Liter bottle of purified water (including for cooking) in one day. When I doubled my water consumption, I lost weight fast.

WHAT IS PURIFIED WATER?
Purified water is being sold in Safeway, Save-On-Foods, Walmart and in many other supermarkets in Canada. Purified water is produced by reverse osmosis or membrane filtration by several US companies such as Primo Water, Culligan and others. Aqua Zone is a Canadian company, selling TWO types of water to businesses and residences throughout the lower mainland of British Columbia, Canada: (i) Spring Water, and (ii) Purified Water

a. Spring Water is produced by a company called "Country Fountain Spring Water Corp" located in Abbotsford, British Columbia, Canada. Spring water is produced from well water (ground water).

b. Purified Water is produced from tap water. They take tap water and further purify it by reducing the TDS (total dissolved solids) level using several techniques in series:
(i) Traditional Filtration (Sedimentation & Activated Carbon Filtration),
(ii) Reverse Osmosis to clean heavy metals, chlorine & fluoride.
(iii) Ultra Violet Radiation (UV Radiaton) to kill the remaining germs.

Primo Water, Culligan, Aqua Zone and many other purified water supply companies use a four-stage water filtration process to turn tap water into purified water, as explained below.

PURIFIED WATER BY REVERSE OSMOSIS (PRIMO WATER) [3]

Tap water is purified to obtain drinkable water by a four-stage filtration process:

1. Sedimentation Filters:
   Reduces particles such as dirt, rust, algae and oxidized iron.
2. Activated Carbon Filters:
Reduces organic taste and odors. Also reduces chlorine taste, earthy moldy, fishy tastes and other odor-causing compounds.
3. Reverse Osmosis: Reverse osmosis reduces dissolved solids and microscopic impurities by forcing water through an ultrafine reverse osmosis membrane. It removes chlorine, fluoride and 98% of all contaminants.
4. Ultraviolet Light: An added final polish, just before vending, ensuring the highest quality water. The contaminants removed or reduced by this process may not necessarily be in the source water.

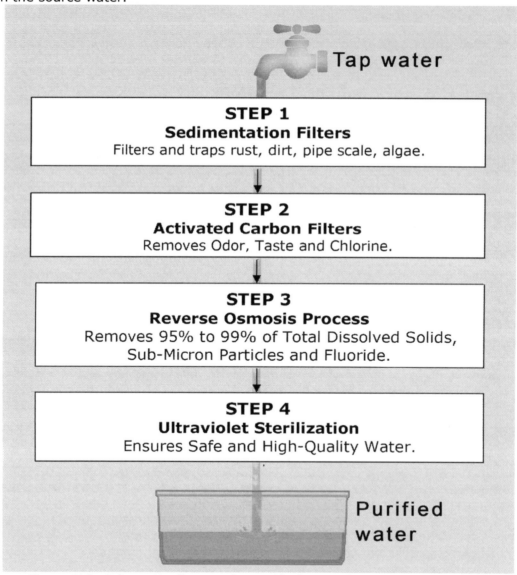

Figure 5.2 Schematic diagram for purified water by reverse osmosis.

How To Know That The Water You Drink Is Indeed Purified?

Do not rely on labels and word of mouth. Purchase your own testing kits and test your drinking water every now and then. The following meter and kit are recommended.
a. TDS meter to Monitor TDS Level (TDS=Total Dissolved Solids) [4]
b. Chlorine Level and Fluoride Level Test Kits (Strips) [5]

If you purchase water purified by reverse osmosis, you don't need to test for chlorine, fluoride and other harmful chemicals. You just test TDS levels, and make sure it is consistently where it is supposed to be. Purified water by Primo Company is supposed to be below 5 ppm. Primo purified water is available in all Safeway and Save-On-Foods stores.

I purchased the following TDS testing meter from Amazon.ca: [4]
HM Digital TDS-4TM Handheld Hydro Tester TDS and Temperature Tester
ASIN # B001RK38LU, PART # HMDIGITALTDS4, Price: $22.60 CAD

https://www.amazon.ca/HM-Digital-TDS-4TM-Handheld-Temperature/dp/B001RK38LU/ref=sr_1_1?ie=UTF8&qid=1437459250&sr=8-1&keywords=TDS-4+Water+Tester+by+HM+Digital

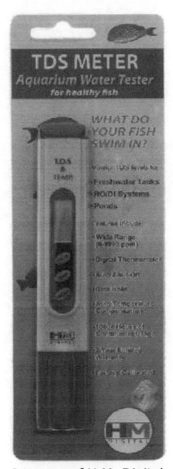

Courtesy of H.M. Digital

Figure 5.3 TDS meter to test the presence of total dissolved solids in water.

After I purchased the aforementioned TDS testing meter, I tested the purified water from Safeway, Save-On-Foods and Walmart to make sure the water is indeed purified.

Listed below are some of the test results I recorded using TDS meter:
29-Jul-2015   I Tested Purified Water from Safeway   TDS=2 ppm
29-Jul-2015   I Tested Purified Water from Save-On-Foods   TDS=4 ppm/3 ppm
29-Jul-2015   I Tested Distilled Water from Walmart   TDS=0 ppm
29-Jul-2015   I Tested Tap Water at my home in Burnaby   TDS=16 ppm

Acceptable TDS Levels for Drinking Water [6, 7]

While different governments set different standards depending on the region, United States EPA sets the standard for TDS level for drinking water as 500 mg/L or 500 ppm.

The World Health Organization (WHO), after conducting a thorough research by a panel of tasters, came up with the following standards for TDS levels in drinking water:

Table 5.1 Acceptable TDS levels for drinking water.

TDS Level (mg/L or ppm)	Rating
< 300 mg/L or ppm	Excellent
300 – 600 mg/L or ppm	Good
600 – 900 mg/L or ppm	Fair
900 – 1200 mg/L or ppm	Poor
> 1200 mg/L or ppm	Unacceptable
	or dangerous

However health experts believe that the TDS levels for ideal drinking water should be under 50 ppm. Even the TDS levels of 50 ppm would be too high for older people with health issues. Therefore health experts recommend that the lesser the TDS level is, the better for older people. That is why the aforementioned companies such as Primo Water, Culligan, Aqua Zone and others have been further purifying tap water using the reverse osmosis membrane filtration technique, and have been lowering the TDS level possibly to 4 ppm or even to 2 ppm. Distilled water has the TDS level of zero ppm.

After conducting my own research, I started buying purified water from Safeway, which has a TDS level of 2 to 4 ppm. Every now and then (every few months), I test the purified water using my TDS meter, and make sure that the water is not contaminated. I also boil purified water using a kettle to make sure any undetected E-coli would be destroyed. Purified and boiled water is then cooled in the fridge before drinking. So I drink purified, boiled and cold water, about 16 cups per day.

BRITA WATER FILTRATION UNIT
BRITA PURIFIED WATER, POSTED BY BRITA.Ca

The Website of Brita Claims that: [8]
Brita® Pitcher filter is packed with activated carbon and ion exchange resin, which work together to filter out the impurities. The carbon in the filter reduces chlorine, while the ion exchange resin reduces metals such as copper, cadmium, mercury and zinc. Brita® claims that the filtered water is healthier and great-tasting.

Brita® Pitcher & Dispenser Water Filters reduce chlorine (taste and odour), copper, mercury, cadmium, zinc and other particulates. Brita® Faucet System Water Filters reduce lead, THMs, VOCs, lindane (pesticide), 2.4-D, alachlor & atrazine (herbicides), chlorine (taste and odour) and particulates. And Brita® Bottles are NSF certified to reduce chlorine (taste and odour) and particulates.

In a Brita® Faucet filter, there is a two-step process: When you turn on your tap, water first passes through a non-woven screen around the filter to trap sediment and particulates. In the 2nd step, the water flows through a compressed block of activated carbon and zeolite, reducing chlorine (taste and odour) and lead.

The Website of Brita Also Claims that: [9]
Brita® Pitcher and Faucet filters are certified under the Water Quality Association (WQA) Gold Seal Product Certification Program. WQA's Gold Seal immediately identifies that Brita® products meet or exceed industry standards for specified contaminant reduction, structural integrity and material safety. Brita® Pitcher and Faucet filters have also been tested and certified by the WQA against NSF/ANSI Standards 42 and 53 for the reduction of the claims specified on the Performance Data Sheet.

The Website of Brita Also Claims that: [10]
While the quality of U.S. and Canadian tap water is generally quite good, chlorine is often added as a disinfectant by certain municipalities, and lead can leach out of household plumbing. Brita® pitcher and faucet water filtration systems reduce the following common impurities, and can even remove 96.6% of pharmaceuticals including Acetaminophen, Carbamazepine, Estradiol, Naproxen and Progesterone. Brita® proudly announces that every time you drink a glass of great-tasting Brita® water, remember you're watering yourself with filtered water that your body truly appreciates.

ZEROWATER FILTRATION UNIT
ZEROWATER PURIFIED WATER, POSTED BY ZEROWATER.Com

The Website of ZeroWater Claims that: [11]
The ZeroWater® Ion Exchange Filter consist of 5 stages that combine patented technologies to removes organic and inorganic contaminants in the water, providing the only filtered water that meets the FDA definition of purified bottled water.

It is a 5 stage filter which is more comprehensive than conventional 2 stage filters. Its Ion Exchange Technology is superior to simple carbon only filters. It removes virtually all (99.6%) detectable dissolved solids while leading brands removes up to 50%.

ZeroWater also claims that: Even if all the municipalities with superior technological advancements achieve the removal of 99.6% of total dissolved solids, the water could pick up chemicals, lead and dirt on its way from the treatment plant, through pipelines, to the faucet. Even the minute quantities of the added chlorine by municipalities is harmful to the children. The taste of the tap water may not be appreciated and the quality may not be trustworthy.

ZeroWater also claims that: Distilled water involves the process of boiling the water in the first container, transferring the steam to another container were the vapors are condensed and everything that doesn't evaporate will remain in the first container. But some impurities could pass through the vapors. That means the impurities that evaporate will be in the water in the second container. While ZeroWater uses the process of deionization which involves filtering the water. The ion exchange beads in the filter takes the ions or minerals out of the water. People usually say that distilled water can taste flat whereas ZeroWater is described as crisp and refreshing. Distillation also requires electricity and takes hours to treat water. Their claim implies that purified water by ZeroWater 5-Stage Fltration System is superior to distilled water.

ZEROWATER 7-CUP WATER FILTRATION ZUG, POSTED BY ZERO WATER.co.uk [12]

The website of Zerowater.co.uk claims that: ZeroWater's 7-cup water filtration jug is designed specifically to fit in standard UK fridge doors and is the first in its class to have a sealed lid and reservoir, making it possible to pour water that has already been filtered without spilling water that's still filtering. This pitcher features an ergonomic, space-saving design perfect for mini-fridges or for users who prefer a lightweight pitcher. The unit purifies the tap water, producing instantly great-tasting water, and the only pour-through filter pitcher on the market that's certified by the NSF to reduce both lead and chromium. ZeroWater filtration jugs also remove 99% of all Fluoride from the tap water.
ZeroWater's first layer of filtration, activated carbon and oxidation reduction alloy removes the chlorine taste you are accustomed to with tap water. The Ion Exchange stage removes virtually all dissolved solids that may be left over from public water systems or even leached into your water from piping such as aluminum, lead, zinc, nitrate and more. Three additional stages are included to remove other impurities and to ensure your water receives the appropriate amount of treatment time to deliver a "000" reading on your water quality meter.

ZEROWATER PURIFIED WATER Vs BRITA PURIFIED WATER [13]
ZeroWater posted the scientific results, comparing the ZeroWater Unit against Brita Unit on how much each unit is capable to filter and eliminate impurities with regards to inorganics, metals, pesticides, and VOC (Volatile Organic Compounds). The website of Zerowater.com claimed that their published data indicate that the ZeroWater filtration system is far superior to the Brita filtration system. Their results can be found on the following webpage:

https://www.zerowater.com/comparison-chart.php

CAN BRITA & ZEROWATER FILTRATION UNITS BE TRUSTED AT HOME (by Blind Faith) TO MAKE PURIFIED WATER FROM TAP WATER?

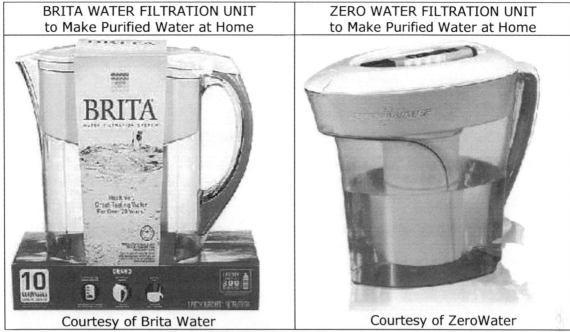

BRITA WATER FILTRATION UNIT to Make Purified Water at Home	ZERO WATER FILTRATION UNIT to Make Purified Water at Home
Courtesy of Brita Water	Courtesy of ZeroWater

Figure 5.4 Water filtration units by Brita and ZeroWater.

My personal experience tells me that these units are unnecessary depending on where you live. You got to be very careful when you buy these units. I did the following experiment to test the Brita filtration unit. I bought the Brita Water filter, and made purified water from tap water. I tested both the tap water and purified water separately by means of a TDS meter, and noted the results carefully. When I tested my tap water, TDS=16 ppm. After I made the purified water using Brita filter, I tested the filtered water. But the filtered water from Brita filter gave me the same result, TDS=16 ppm, which obviously means Brita filter does not filter the total dissolved solids (TDS) of the tap water in the area where I live (Burnaby, British Columbia, Canada). So I did not trust Brita filter and decided not to use it.

I then decided to buy purified water from Safeway. The reverse osmosis unit (by PRIMO WATER) that they have in Safeway, Save-On-Foods, and other supermarkets filters the tap water and reduces total dissolved solids (TDS) concentration from 16 ppm to 4 ppm or even to 2 ppm. I also tested the purified water (by reverse osmosis) from Safeway, and it gave me TDS =4 ppm. I concluded that the purified water from Safeway is trustworthy.

Maybe, Brita filter lowers TDS from 500 ppm to 200 ppm or from 200 ppm to 100 ppm, but does not lower TDS from 16 ppm to 2 ppm. Brita filters could be beneficial in cities where the water is contaminated by having very high TDS levels 300 ppm, 500 ppm or 1000 ppm, but it is unnecessary in municipalities where the water is already purified. After this experience with Brita filtration unit, I did not test the ZeroWater filtration unit, and preferred to purchase purified water by reverse osmosis being sold in Safeway, Save-On-Foods, and other grocery stores.

RECOMMENDATION

Do not purchase and use Brita Filtration Unit or ZeroWater Filtration Unit by relying on blind faith or word of mouth. After you purchase any of these units, test it by means of a TDS meter. Monitor the TDS values of both tap water and filtered water, and compare the results. If the Brita Filtration Unit or ZeroWater Fltration Unit does not filter tap water by lowering the TDS value significantly, that means the unit is unnecessary, you better return it and get the money back. If the unit lowers TDS value of tap water significantly, then you keep the unit and use it for your drinking water.

HOW DRINKING WATER SPEEDS UP WEIGHT LOSS?

Drinking Water May Speed Weight Loss [14]
Researchers in Germany Found That Drinking Lots of Water May Speed Up Weight Loss; Metabolic Rate Increases Slightly With An Increase in Water Consumption
After drinking approximately 17 ounces (2 cups) of water, the subjects' metabolic rates increased by 30% for both men and women.

How Does Water Flush Fat Out of Your System? [15]
Drinking water before you eat may help you eat less. A 2010 study published on Obesity investigated the effects of drinking 2 cups of water before meals on weight loss among a group of people following a low-calorie diet. The study found that the water-drinking group lost more weight than the control group. Drinking water before you eat helps fill you up so you eat less, which may help you lose weight.

Does Water Flush Out Fat? (Discussion Forum) [16]
Water flushes out fat cells and ketones. Hydration is extremely important for this and it also keeps our bowels working correctly. Water also flushes out water weight. It sounds stupid and does not make sense, but some of our weight is in water and by drinking water we flush out that old water weight that is sticking onto us and you actually may lose a few pounds after drinking water.

Whether you are dieting or not, water consumption is essential for good health. You're not flushing out fat cells, but rather flushing out the waste products your body makes. You are right about water retention, the body tends to hold onto water if there isn't enough coming in.

Water: How 8 Glasses A Day Keep Fat Away? [17, 18]
Drinking Enough Water is the Best Treatment for Fluid Retention.
Water is needed in great quantities for fat metabolism and for the disposal of waste generated once fats are metabolized. When a person is obese or overweight, he/she needs more water than he/she would require with normal body weight. Water flushes away the waste. When a person loses weight (losing weight means burning fat), the body becomes very busy getting rid of a lot of waste generated due to fat metabolism.

When water retention becomes a serious problem, you need to cut salt consumption. When you consume excess salt, your body retains more and more water to dilute the sodium. If you want to get rid of excess sodium in your system, drink plenty of water. As water is forced through the kidneys, it will remove the excess sodium.

When you drink limited quantity of water, the body perceives that there is scarcity of water for future survival, and begins to store water in the extracellular spaces, outside the cell walls. This kind of water storage could cause swollen feet, swollen legs and swollen hands. Doctors then prescribe diuretics to their patients to force out the stored water from the extracellular spaces. But if you drink plenty of water (at least 8 glasses per day), you would not encounter such situations. Drinking plenty of water also helps constipation.

The Water Report: [19]
How 8 Glasses of Water per Day Fights Weight Gain!

Pure and clean water may be the only true Magic Potion for permanent weight loss!
If you stop drinking enough water your body fluids will again be thrown out of balance.

DRINKING ICE-COLD WATER BURNS MORE CALORIES: Cold water is absorbed more quickly into the system than warm water. Evidence suggests that by drinking ice-cold water a person can actually burn more calories. In order to raise the ice-cold water temperature to your normal body temperature (normal body temperature is 37°C/98.6°F), your body has to work hard and burn more calories.

When the body gets enough water to function optimally, all the body system fluids will achieve perfect balance. As a result, the endocrine gland function improves, fluid retention is alleviated as stored water is lost, more fat can be used as fuel because the liver is free to metabolize stored fat, natural thirst to drink water returns, and there is a loss of hunger almost overnight.

DRINKING LOTS OF WATER REDUCES FAT DEPOSITS: Kidneys cannot function properly without drinking enough water. When the kidneys do not function, the liver takes responsibility to do the kidney's job. But the liver's primary function is to metabolize stored fat into usable energy for the body. But if the liver has to do some of the kidney's work, it cannot work at full throttle. So you must drink lots of water to help your body.

DRINK PURIFIED WATER: Environmental Protection Agency (EPA) began enforcing the water purification and treatment standards for municipal water systems long ago. But there continues to be incidents of contamination, which could be harmful to your health. So you cannot trust tap water even if your local municipality says that the tap water is being purified. You take your own measures to make sure that the water you drink is indeed purified. Installing your own water filtration system at home would be the best option.

However, you should monitor the purified water every now and then and make sure the water is not contaminated. You can do that by using a TDS meter to test the purified water as explained above.

What 8 Cups of Water Per Day Would Do To Your Body?
How Drinking Water Would Help Improve Your Overall Health?

- Increases metabolism (cold water).
- Makes you feel full (warm water).
- Helps you lose weight.
- Flushes out toxins.
- Gets you healthier skin.
- Reduces risk of certain cancers.
- Helps digestion and constipation.
- Relieves fatigue and energizes.
- Improves overall health.
- All of the above for ZERO calories.

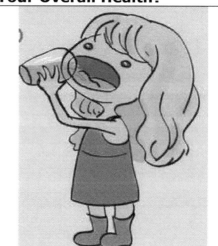

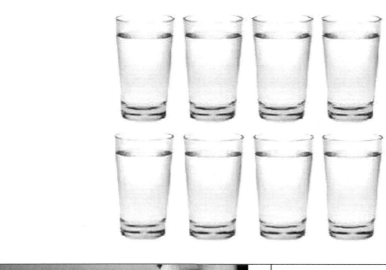

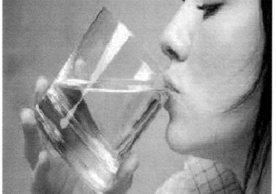

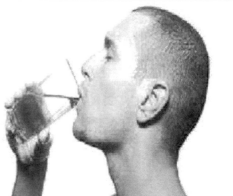

Figure 5.5 How drinking water would help improve your overall health.

REFERENCES

1. Hydration: Why It Is Important by FamilyDoctor.Org.
   https://familydoctor.org/hydration-why-its-so-important/

2. Benefits of Water by Brita.ca.
https://brita.ca/water-wellness/benefits/

3. Brochures being distributed by Primo® Water (Primowater.com) and Culligan® Water (Culliganwater.com).
https://primowater.com/
https://www.culligan.com/home

4. HM Digital TDS-4TM Handheld Hydro Tester TDS and Temperature Tester ASIN # B001RK38LU, PART # HMDIGITALTDS4, Price: $22.60 CAD.
https://www.amazon.ca/HM-Digital-TDS-4TM-Handheld-Temperature/dp/B001RK38LU/ref=sr_1_1?ie=UTF8&qid=1437459250&sr=8-1&keywords=TDS-4+Water+Tester+by+HM+Digital

5. Chlorine & Fluoride Test Kits.
   http://www.microwaterman.com/TestingKits/FluorideTestKit.html

6. What is the acceptable TDS level of drinking water?
   https://www.quora.com/What-is-the-acceptable-TDS-level-of-drinking-water

7. Drinking Water Standards.
   http://www.tdsmeter.com/education?id=0018

8. Brita Water Filtration Unit by Brita.ca, How It Works?, Posted by Brita.ca
https://brita.ca/water-filtration-process/

9. Benefits of Brita Filtered Water, Posted by Brita.ca.
https://brita.ca/water-wellness/benefits/

10. Water Quality and Contaminants, Posted by Brita.ca.
https://brita.ca/water-filtration-process/water-quality-contamination/

11. ZeroWater Filtration Unit: How It Works?
https://www.zerowater.com/faq-how-does-it-work.php

12. 7-CUP ZEROWATER WATER FILTRATION JUG.
https://zerowater.co.uk/products/zerowater-7-cup-1-66-litre-water-filtrater-jug?gclid=Cj0KCQiAvrfSBRC2ARIsAFumcm8DOn4CC1af0ThgEKewd6I_-zYerKiLsDuYwouWBNP3jnT9yZF5Oz4aApMUEALw_wcB

13. Comparison of Zero Water Unit and Brita Unit, Posted by ZeroWater.
https://www.zerowater.com/comparison-chart.php

14. Drinking Water May Speed Weight Loss by WebMD.com.
   http://www.webmd.com/diet/news/20040105/drinking-water-may-speed-weight-loss

15. How Does Water Flush Fat Out of Your System? by JILL CORLEONE, RDN, LD Last Updated: Jun 17, 2015.
  http://www.livestrong.com/article/545311-how-does-water-flush-fat-out-of-your-system/

16. Does Water Flush Out Fat? (Discussion Forum).
  http://forum.lowcarber.org/archive/index.php/t-336946.html

17. Water: How 8 Glasses A Day Keep Fat Away by Angelfire.com.
  http://www.angelfire.com/ca2/LowcarbingDream/water.html

18. The Snowbird Diet by Donald S. Roberston, M.D., M. Sc., A Book Published by Donald S. Robertson, MD on Amazon.com.
https://www.amazon.com/snowbird-diet-slender-future-lifetime/dp/0446382833

19. The Water Report: How 8 Glasses of Water per Day Fights Weight Gain! by Colon Therapists Network.
  http://www.colonhealth.net/healtharticles/8-glasses-water-per-day-fights-weight-gain.html

CHAPTER 6 BODY MASS INDEX (BMI)

TABLE OF CONTENTS

BODY MASS INDEX (BMI)

WHAT IS BODY MASS INDEX?
Body mass index (BMI) is a measure of body fat based on height and weight that applies to adult men and women. [1, 3, 4]

BMI was first proposed for obesity studies by Adolphe Quetelet, a Belgian astronomer, mathematician, statistician and sociologist during 1830 to 1850. [3, 4] The definition of BMI, as the ratio of human body weight to the height squared, was later published by Ancel Keys in the July 1972 edition of the Journal of Chronic Diseases. [3] Ancel Keys reported that BMI can be used as an indicator of relative obesity.

National Heart, Lung and Blood Institute (NHLBI) and National Institute of Diabetes and Digestive and Kidney Diseases (NIDDK) released the following obesity guidelines: [1, 5, 6]

(i) A Body Mass Index (BMI) value equal to or greater than 30 indicates OBESITY
(ii) A Body Mass Index (BMI) value between 25 and 29.9 indicates OVERWEIGHT
(iii) A Body Mass Index (BMI) value between 18.5 and 24.9 corresponds to NORMAL
(iv) A Body Mass Index (BMI) value below 18.5 indicates UNDERWEIGHT

The following table shows the same guidelines:

Table 6.1 Assessment Guidelines for Body Mass Index.

BMI	Assessment
Below 18.5	Underweight
18.5 – 24.9	Normal Body Weight
25.0 – 29.9	Overweight
30.0 and Above	Obese

FORMULA TO CALCULATE BODY MASS INDEX
The following formula has been universally accepted to calculate BMI: [4]

BMI Formula in Metric Units (UK)	BMI Formula in Imperial Units (USA)
$$BMI = \frac{(\text{weight in kilograms})}{\text{height in meters}^2}$$	$$BMI = \frac{(\text{weight in pounds} \times 703)}{\text{height in inches}^2}$$

Figure 6.1 Body mass index formula.

HOW TO CALCULATE BODY MASS INDEX?
HOW TO CALCULATE THE EXCESS BODY WEIGHT YOU HAVE?

Body Mass Index (BMI) is calculated in metric units as follows: [1]

$$BMI = Weight\ (Kg) / [Height\ (m)]^2$$

- If the weight is known in pounds, convert to Kg.
- If the height is known in feet and inches, convert to meters.
- Substitute the values in the formula, and then calculate the BMI.

Conversion Factors
1 Kg = 2.2222 Pounds; 1 Pound = 0.45 Kg
1 Meter = 3.281 Feet = 39.37 Inches
1 Foot = 0.3048 Meter
1 Inch = 0.0254 Meter

Sample Calculation of BMI
George is 5′ 6″ tall and currently weighs 190 pounds (lb). How many pounds should George lose to lower his body mass index (BMI) to normal?

Height = 5′ 6″ = 66 Inches = (66)(0.0254) = 1.6764 m
Weight = 190 lb = (190/2.2222) = 85.50 Kg
BMI = $(85.50)/(1.6764)^2$ = 30.42   Assessment = Obese

Sample Calculation of Excess Body Weight
a. Find out your weight in Kg (1 Kg = 2.2222 lb).
b. Find out your height in meters (1 meter = 3.281 feet = 39.37 inches).
c. For a normal BMI of less than or equal to 24.9, what would be your weight?
d. Calculate your normal weight (Kg) by substituting the values in the formula.
e. By knowing your current weight (Kg), and your normal weight that you just
   calculated, find out the excess body weight you have.

For a healthy weight, let us suppose reasonably that the BMI should be equal to or less than 24.5. So George's goal should be to lower his BMI from 30.29 to 24.5. Using the aforementioned formula for BMI, the weight that corresponds to a BMI of 24.5 is calculated as follows:

BMI   = Weight (Kg) / $[Height\ (m)]^2$
24.5   = Weight (Kg)/ $[1.68]^2$
Therefore Weight in Kg   = (24.5) multiplied by $[1.6764]^2$
     = (24.5) (1.68)(1.68)
     = 68.85 Kg (which is the normal weight)

So the Excess Weight of George = 85.50 – 68.85 = 16.65 Kg = 36.99 lb
That means George should lose at least 16.65 Kg or 37 pounds to lower his Body Mass Index (BMI) to normal.

If you have difficulty of doing calculations or if you don't like calculations at all, then use the following website of National Heart, Lung and Blood Institute to find out your body mass index (BMI): [6]

https://www.nhlbi.nih.gov/health/educational/lose_wt/BMI/bmicalc.htm
You simply enter your weight (pounds) and height (feet, inches) , it will calculate BMI for you.

LIMITATIONS OF THE BMI FORMULA [4]

The BMI formula has been criticized by many health and fitness experts as it does not suit every body type. The formula fits well only for adults with the regular body type. The BMI formula is not suitable for:

a. Body builders who intentionally build big muscles
b. Shorter people though their bodies are grown to maturity
c. Pregnant and lactating women
d. Children whose bodies are not yet grown to maturity
e. Elderly people whose muscle mass reduces with age

BODY FAT PERCENTAGE

If the BMI formula does not suit your body type, then find out your body fat percentage using the body fat analyzer. This unit calculates your body fat percentage with a reasonable degree of accuracy. Any body fat percentage that is lower than 24.5% or even 25% is considered normal. You should lose weight until your body fat percentage is normal.

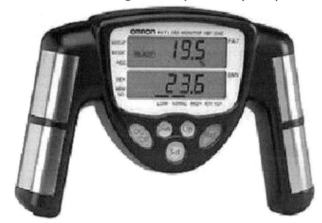

Courtesy of Omron Corp.
Figure 6.2 Omron body fat analyzer (Model HBF-306).

Body fat percentage can also be determined by calipers method or through the use of bioelectrical impedance analysis.

WAIST CIRCUMFERENCE

The measurement of waist circumference is another indicative of body fat. When you have excess body fat and thus excess body weight, your waist circumstance grows to an unacceptable level. In such cases, you must take immediate action to lower your waist circumference to normal. Each adult person has his/her own normal waist ranging from 30 inches to 34 inches, depending on the height of the person.

If your Body Mass Index (BMI) is normal or if your body fat percentage is normal, your waist would automatically look normal. If you have excess body weight or excess body fat, your waist would automatically look abnormal.

According to the US National Institutes of Health (NIH), a waist circumference in excess of 40 inches (or 102 centimeters) for men and a waist circumstance in excess of 35 inches (88 centimeters) for women poses high risk, and could cause type 2 diabetes, dyslipidemia, high blood pressure and several other health concerns. [3]

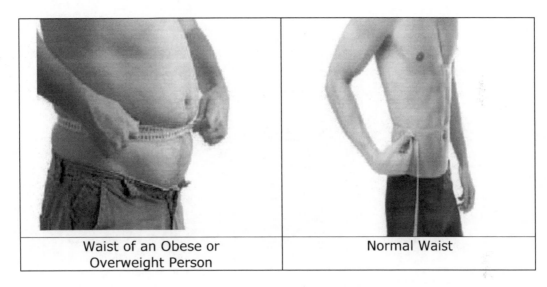

Waist of an Obese or Overweight Person	Normal Waist

Figure 6.3 Waist circumference of obese person and normal person.

BY LOWERING THE BODY MASS INDEX (BMI), YOU CAN ATTAIN YOUR WEIGHT-LOSS GOAL

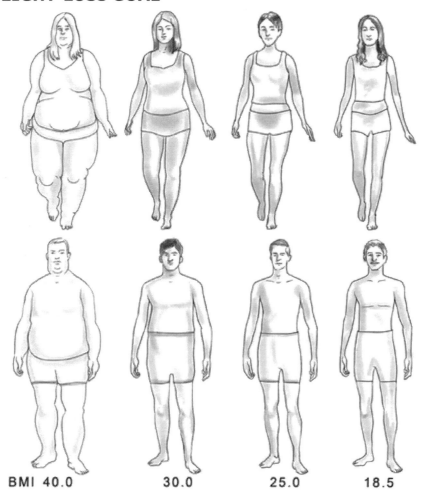

BMI 40.0   30.0   25.0   18.5

Figure 6.4 The drop of body mass index from obese person to normal person.

A body mass index (BMI) of 25 or below 25 is considered normal. So an obese person or overweight person should lose weight by monitoring his/her BMI every week until their BMI reaches 25 or below. In the picture shown above, an obese person's body mass index (BMI) gradually dropped from 40 to 18.5, which is perfectly normal.

How Dr. RK Lowered His BMI to Normal

Dr. RK lowered his BMI from 30.5 to 24 in 22 months. He accomplished this result by eating whole foods, by avoiding processed foods (See his Weight-Loss Diet Level-II explained in the main article), daily exercise, and with high willpower and high self-discipline. By lowering the BMI to perfectly normal, he successfully reversed his obesity and obstructive sleep apnea.

If you understand how to monitor the BMI once every week, and follow the instructions outlined in the weight-loss course (see main article), you can very easily lose weight and maintain a normal body weight and normal BMI for the rest of your life.

REFERENCES

1. Permanent Diabetes Control, Authored by Rao Konduru, PhD, Reviewed and Endorsed by Dr. Marshall Dahl, MD, PhD, Page: 51.

2. Website www.mydiabetescontrol.com about Permanent Diabetes Control.

3. Body Mass Index (BMI) from Wikipedia.
https://en.wikipedia.org/wiki/Body_mass_index

4. The BMI Formula in Metric Units (UK) and Imperial Units (USA).
http://www.whathealth.com/bmi/formula.html

5. Calculate Body Mass Index, National Heart, Lung and Blood Institute.
https://www.nhlbi.nih.gov/health/educational/wecan/healthy-weight-basics/body-mass-index.htm

6. Body Mass Index Calculator, National Heart, Lung and Blood Institute.
https://www.nhlbi.nih.gov/health/educational/lose_wt/BMI/bmicalc.htm

About the Author

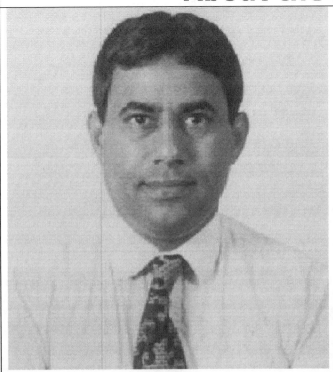

Rao Konduru, PhD (also called Dr. RK) published a book in the past titled "Permanent Diabetes Control", which earned immense respect and appreciation. Many people said it was a wonderful book. After suffering from a sudden heart attack, even though his left artery was 75% clogged and he could not walk a block due to severe angina pain, Dr. RK said "NO" to bypass surgery. He did what none of us would even think of doing. He simply relied on his natural self-prevention diet and exercise, and with it "reversed his critical diabetic heart disease in a matter of months", and developed a method to accomplish Permanent Diabetes Control. He proved to the medical community that a bypass surgery is unnecessary in most cases. He also came up with a trial and error procedure to determine the optimal insulin dose that would tightly control diabetes in 90 days, and would allow a diabetic person to live like a normal person for the rest of his/her life.

Please visit www.mydiabetescontrol.com, and read through the testimonials. Click on the Abstract button to see his official blood test results. Notice the fact that he maintained his hemoglobin A1c levels under 6% consistently. His personal best hemoglobin A1c level of 5% is an extraordinary result any diabetic person would hope to accomplish in a lifetime. Perhaps he is the only diabetic person living in this world now with "Permanent Diabetes Control".

Once again, quite recently health demons, such as uncontrollable weight gain, sleep apnea and chronic insomnia, came his way. Dr. RK did not give up, but persisted on discovering new, natural and effortless treatments of his own in reversing these most difficult disorders, through extensive reading, research, commitment, self-discipline and the strong desire to succeed. His extensive scientific research experience and his powerful knowledge helped him battle and combat these life challenges. He figured out their root causes, and developed natural yet powerful techniques to cure these health disorders. After losing 40 pounds of weight and 12 inches around the waist, Dr. RK successfully reversed his obesity, obstructive sleep apnea and chronic insomnia. He has carefully outlined and illustrated the methods he developed in three excellent books "Reversing Obesity, Reversing Sleep Apnea and Reversing Insomnia", so that others can benefit and be inspired to achieve similar results.
- Prime Publishing Co.

Order your books here:
www.reversingobesity.ca
www.reversingsleepapnea.com
www.reversinginsomnia.com

THE END OF THE "REVERSING OBESITY" COURSE!